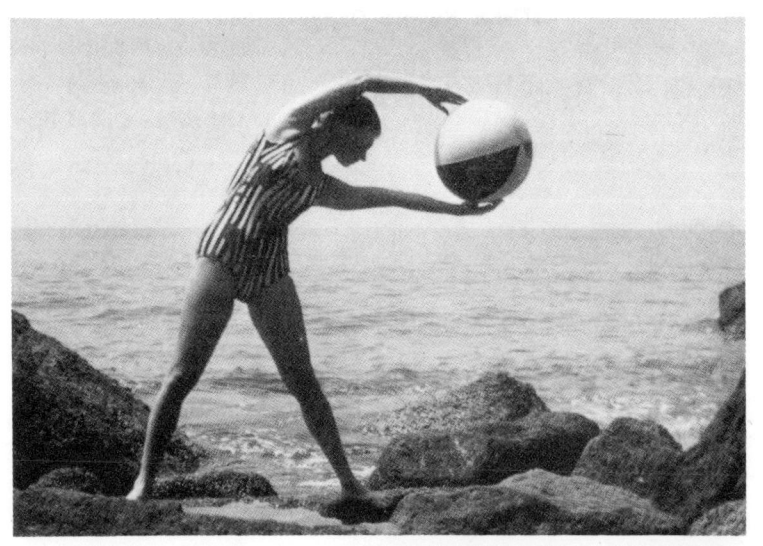

EXERCISE for SPORTS

By Hannelore Pilss-Samek

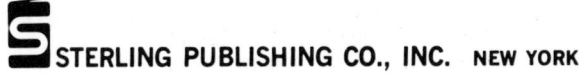
STERLING PUBLISHING CO., INC. NEW YORK

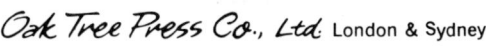
Oak Tree Press Co., Ltd. London & Sydney

OTHER BOOKS OF INTEREST

Advanced Tennis	Getting Started in Tennis
Basketball the Modern Way	Ride a Horse
Bike-Ways	Swimming the Shane Gould Way

ATHLETIC INSTITUTE SERIES

Baseball	Gymnastics
Basketball	Table Tennis
Girls' Basketball	Tumbling and Trampolining
Girls' Gymnastics	Wrestling

Copyright © 1973 by Sterling Publishing Co., Inc.
419 Park Avenue South, New York, N.Y. 10016
British edition published by Oak Tree Press Co., Ltd., Nassau, Bahamas
Distributed in Australia and New Zealand by Oak Tree Press Co., Ltd.,
P.O. Box 34, Brickfield Hill, Sydney 2000, N.S.W.
Distributed in the United Kingdom and elsewhere in the British Commonwealth
by Ward Lock Ltd., 116 Baker Street, London W 1
Originally published under the title "Gymnastik—jederzeit und überall"
Copyright 1966 by Leopold Stocker Verlag, Graz
Manufactured in the United States of America   *All rights reserved*
Library of Congress Catalog Card No.: 73-83461
ISBN 0-8069-4062-X   UK 7061-2475-8
4063-8

CONTENTS

Before You Begin 5
Slenderizing Your Hips 7
Away with Tummy Bulge! 8
For a Willowy Waist 10
Away with That Swayback! 12
For Firm Breasts 14
Stand Up and Be Counted! 16
Firming Flabby Thighs 17
For Naturally Slender Figures 19
Daily Exercising 20
If You Sit All Day 23
If You Stand All Day 25
Relaxation 30
Exercises Especially for the Sportsman 32
Better Posture 38
Tank Up on Fresh Air 44
Travelling with Children 49
Conditioning for the Slopes 53
Practice on the Snow 59
Conditioning for Tennis 67
Beach Exercises 71
A Little Self-Massage 78
Roll Yourself Slim 86
A Final Word 88
Index 95

BEFORE YOU BEGIN

Exercise makes you stronger and slimmer, releases your tensions, and tunes up your body for participation in any sport as well as the game of life.

Not all movement of legs, arms, shoulders and torso can be called exercise, however, nor does it have the same effect. Also exercise without regularity is not as effective as a daily routine.

In this book, you will find many different exercises which can be performed anywhere without special equipment. If you follow them you will train your body properly. If you breathe correctly, walk properly and exercise daily, you should not be overweight or flabby, even if your work is sedentary and you never play any physical games.

But if you are training for a sport, follow all the exercises and particularly the special exercises given here and you will find yourself more alert and ready to play than if you went into the game cold. Your nerves will be less tense, and this means your muscles will be more fluid and responsive to mental signals.

Exercise is not to be taken like cod liver oil. You must enjoy it, and the sports you prepare for through exercise should be played with zest. The game itself, in which you compete or strain to perform at your best, is also a form of exercise — perhaps the best, for you get involved emotionally to such an extent that tension over other things disappears. you concentrate on making your body behave as you play the game — and that is exactly what you intend to achieve with all exercise.

So play joyfully and exercise joyfully. If you don't enjoy bending and stretching, tensing and untensing your body, moving in supple ways rhythmically, then you are not exercising properly.

Let's start with our first movement, which is intended to make your hips slender.

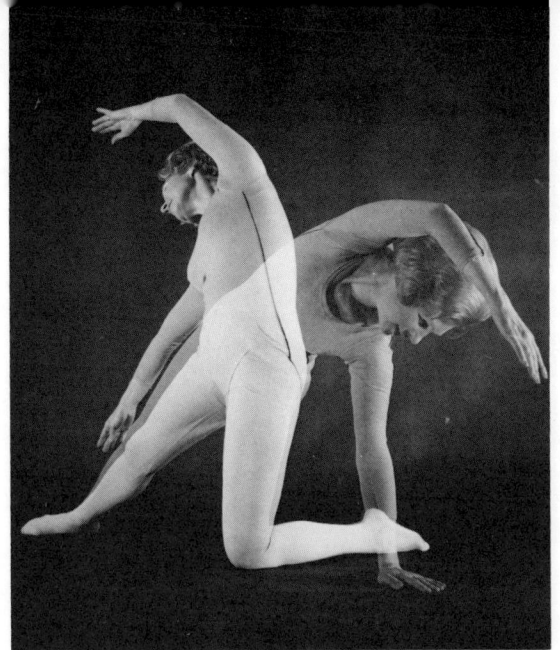

EXERCISE 1:
Bend your torso this way and that way until your hips slim down.

SLENDERIZING YOUR HIPS

Unless you do something about it, fat settles in and remains stubbornly on your hips. Most of us pursue a sedentary way of life that makes it easy for a cushion of fat to develop precisely where you are most often relaxed. One way to exercise is to run in circles. Another is to massage your hips, even if you have to do it yourself. Or you can "roll yourself slim" (see page 86). But probably the best way to get a sporty and elegant figure with slim hips is to try exercise!

Exercise 1: Bend your torso while on your left knee with right leg stretched sideways. Bend twice in the direction of your outstretched leg, inhaling at the same time. Then bend twice in the opposite direction, away from your outstretched leg, supporting yourself on your left hand and exhaling. Practice this four times, then reverse your position, resting on your right knee, left leg outstretched, and repeat the exercise.

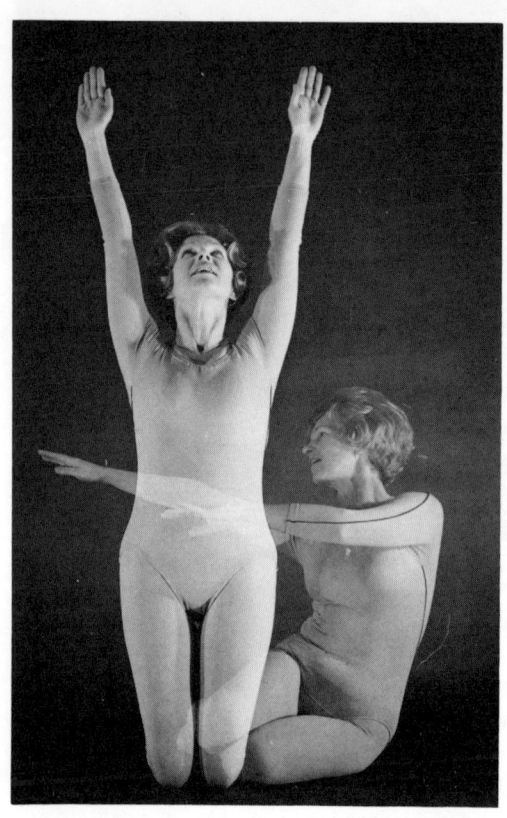

EXERCISE 2:
Down on your knees, but tummy and arms erect. Then sit quickly and swing your arms vigorously until you swing up on your knees again.

AWAY WITH TUMMY BULGE!

The frail sex can take some kind of comfort from the fact that men have to struggle against the tummy bulge evil the same as they do.

More movement! That's what's necessary. If your job keeps you practically motionless all day, you must practice compensating gymnastics. If you travel around a great deal by car, you will also have to offset the lack of bodily movement with exercise. The right approach is to carry heavy packages with both hands (men carried out ashes in the days of coal furnaces) and observing fruit days to help against the bulges brought on by comfortable living. Massage is also good.

Not only do you want to lose weight, but at the same time you must firm up your stomach muscles. Exercise 2 will work not only towards a good figure but also towards good health. The stomach muscles give your body support, much like a girdle made of muscle, and make possible the correct pelvic position, even during heavy exertion. Not least, exercise is an aid to counter a bulging tummy that is caused by indigestion. Let intensive training begin!

Here it is! **Exercise 2:** Sit erect on your knees, and hold your arms up high! Now let yourself down quickly to the left to a sitting position, with most of your weight on your left hip and thigh. Make a counterswing of your arms towards the right and exhale. Now swing your arms vigorously upward and come erect on your knees; inhale. Now sit down to the right and repeat the exercise.

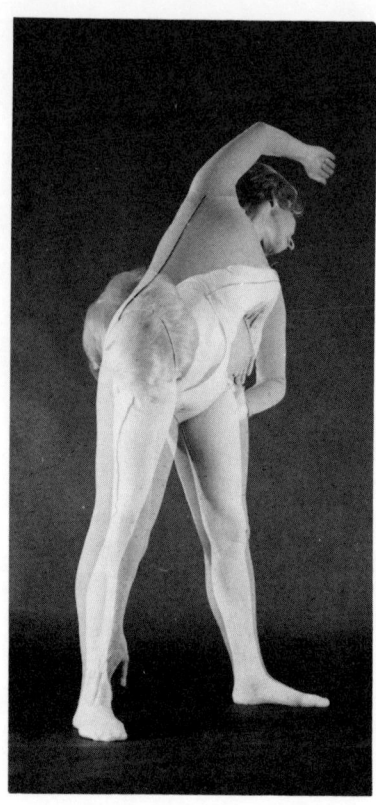

EXERCISE 3:
Feet apart, hand on hip, swing your other arm over your head, and bend. Back up and touch your toe.

FOR A WILLOWY WAIST

The slim waist has always been an especially feminine attribute, as it still is today, but today, too, men are watching their waistlines just as carefully!

Shudder all you want at the iron plates that were worn hundreds of years ago and pity our grandmothers who, seizing the bedpost for support, let themselves be laced up tighter and tighter. Dresses were cut to fit the figure of the wearer, but the poor creatures squeezed their bodies into the proper shape to fit their clothes! It's no wonder that fainting fits were the order of the day.

In those days, it was possible to acquire a slim waist simply by corseting as tightly as necessary, but who can wear a corset in a bikini? A reasonable amount of proper exercise will make you not only slim but willowy. Nonetheless, a slim waist alone won't help you win a tennis match if you are stiff and all your movements are wooden. For slimming as well as flexibility in the waist, try this:

Exercise 3: Stand with feet apart, left hand on your hip. Swing your right arm over your head to the left, bend deeply to the side, spring back, and inhale. Bend down twice to touch your right foot and exhale. Do this four times; then put the other hand on your other hip and repeat on the other side.

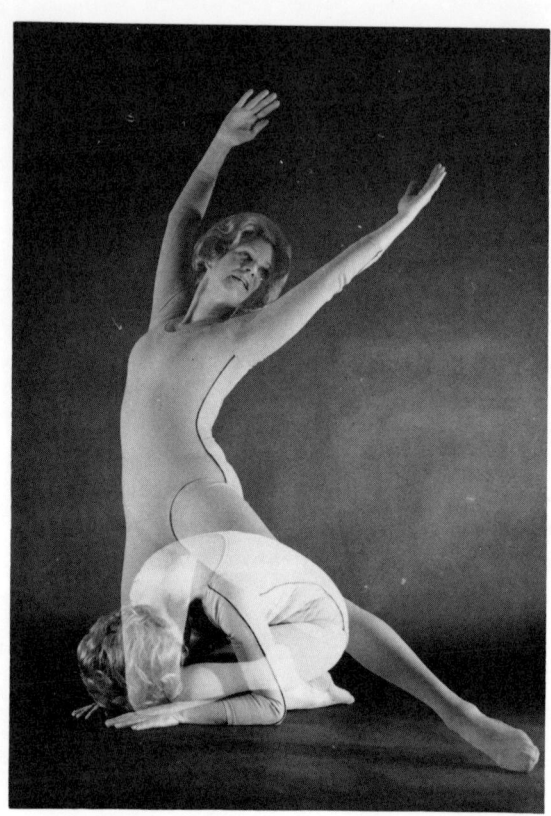

EXERCISE 4:
Curl over, back rounded and exhale. Come up quickly on one knee, other leg out, and inhale.

AWAY WITH THAT SWAYBACK!

The line of the back should be as straight as possible. What good is a slim figure if, from the side, it looks like a question mark? How does this unattractive posture come about? Owing to muscle weakness or laziness, the pelvis sags to the rear, at the same time thrusting its upper edge forward, causing an unhealthy pelvic position. The proper exercises for the back region should make it flexible and strong. A swayback is not only unpleasant, it can be the cause of backache. When you have to stand for long periods of time, avoid letting your pelvis sag backwards. This is usually the first reaction when feet get tired. With a little stretching of your tummy muscles and those at the bottom of your pelvis, your pelvis can remain in the natural and correct position, and overtiring of the back region is avoided unless you have a swayback! Get rid of it by working on this exercise:

Exercise 4: On your knees, sit on your heels and curl over. Round your back, and exhale. Snap quickly erect on your right knee, left leg thrust to the side, arms and torso inclined towards the thrust-out leg. Inhale. Now, back to the starting position; exhale. On the next swing up, thrust your other leg to the side.

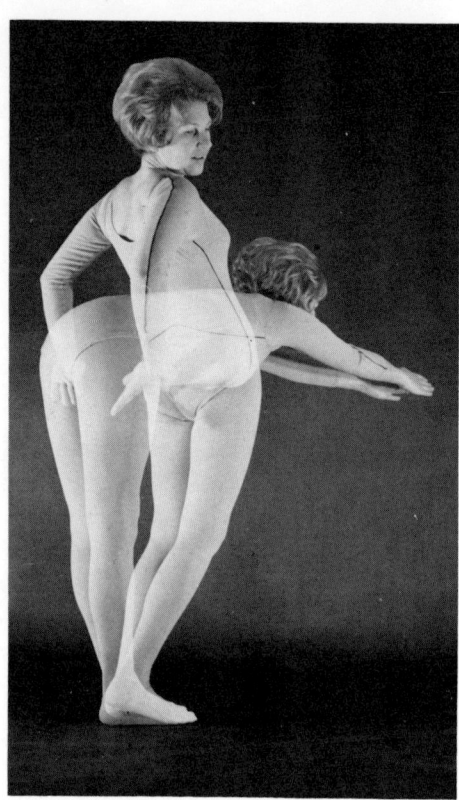

EXERCISE 5:
Bend over and reach out, exhaling. Up again, swing arms back, and inhale.

FOR FIRM BREASTS

There are sundry preparations available that guarantee women a completely beautiful bust after only a short period of use. Emollients on the outside and pills on the inside are supposed to work wonders simultaneously. But firming of the glands alone does not guarantee success — posture and firmness of the breast muscles must take first place.

A word on breast care: Douche the breasts every morning with a stream of cold water. If you have no douching apparatus, bend over the basin and splatter cold water with your hand from beneath. This will also stimulate the circulation. Massage only the breast muscle, that is, the muscle leading from the shoulder to the breast. With your right hand, take the left muscle between your thumb and your remaining fingers, gripping deeply and thoroughly kneading. Massage the right with your left hand. Don't wear a brassiere that is too tight. Such constriction throughout an entire day will never allow the breast muscles to function on their own. Try as many firming exercises as you can during the course of the day, such as kneading dough, window cleaning, lifting, boosting things up, playing tennis, badminton or golf and, expecially, swimming.

Now try this. **Exercise 5:** Feet together, bend forward, stretch out your arms and bring your palms together, at the same time exhaling. Then straighten up, push your knees forward, swing your arms backwards and again press your palms together behind your back. Inhale!

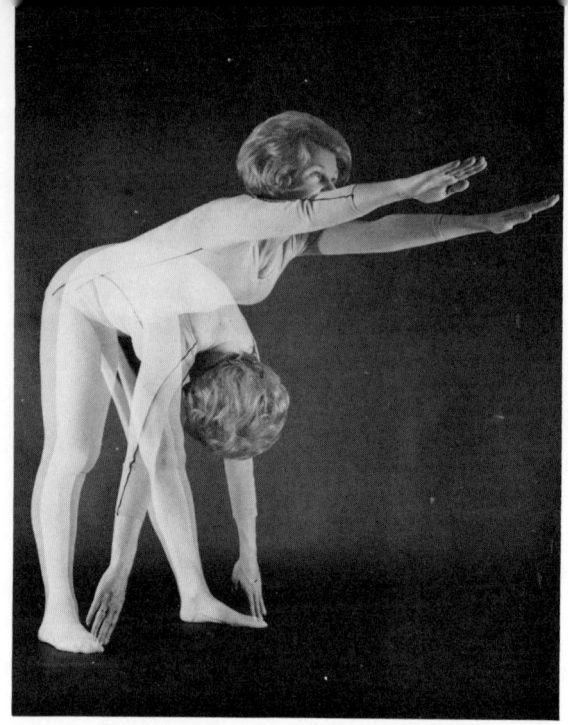

EXERCISE 6:
Hang over, relaxed. Raise up slowly and inhale. Back down, relax, and exhale.

STAND UP AND BE COUNTED!

Good posture doesn't mean "chest out" and your lungs expanded! A perfect posture can overcome many figure defects since it is important for the entire figure. Don't just stand aside, resigned and depressed. Make use of exercise!

A perfect carriage does not begin with the shoulders, but with the position of the pelvis. It is also a matter of stretching abdominal and lower pelvic muscles, so that the pelvis cannot sag off backwards into a swayback position. The whole body is stretched, the head held naturally high, and there should be no double chin. Now, begin the exercise!

Exercise 6: Legs apart, knees stiff, let your torso hang down relaxed. Now slowly raise your trunk to horizontal, head high. Inhale. Take the beginning position again. Exhale.

EXERCISE 7:
Going from a hanging position to a standing position will do wonders for your upper leg tone.

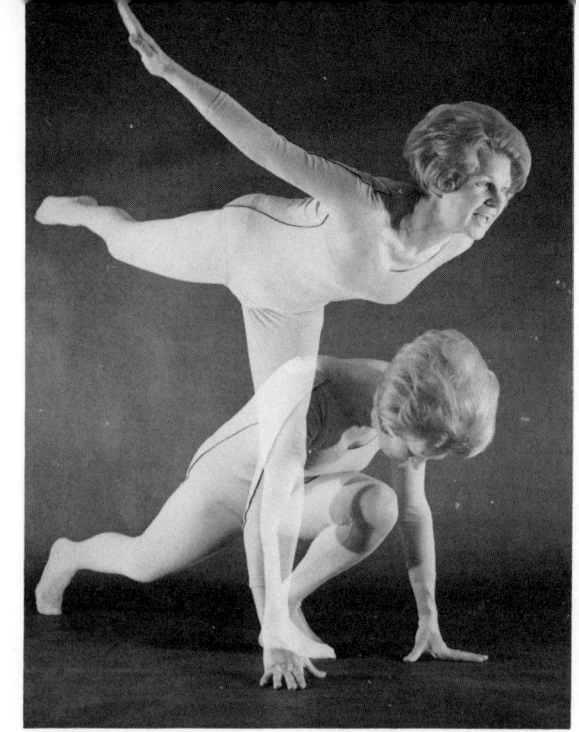

FIRMING FLABBY THIGHS

Even if you have well shaped thighs, exercise can help them to look even better and stay that way. Flabby thighs are one of the first signs of approaching age!

Go short distances on foot — long standing spells trouble for legs; they will swell and hurt. On the other hand, active walking involves not only the legs but also the entire body. Your muscles will become firm, especially those of the thighs. Try a little self-massage every day on your thighs. Simplest is a brush massage using a dry, medium-hard brush, as well as strong kneading with both hands. (For more on self-massage, see page 77.) This exercise will be a boon for bicycle riders, among others. Here it is:

Exercise 7: Racing position with the right leg stretched out

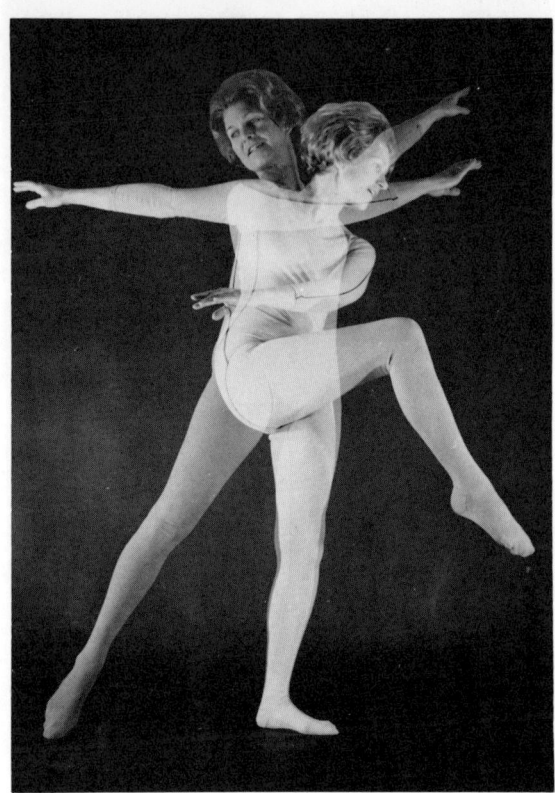

EXERCISE 8:
Stretch your leg to the side and raise your arms. Then lift and point your knee to the opposite side. Swing your arms across your knee.

behind, supporting yourself with both hands on the floor. Lower yourself twice, bending your elbows. Then quickly up, arms out to the sides; straighten the standing leg; inhale. Again drop down, deep bend; exhale. Repeat four times, then do the exercise on your other leg.

FOR NATURALLY SLENDER FIGURES

Who doesn't envy those who can eat whatever they please without the slightest little pad of fat resulting! Worry about their figures and calorie tables does not seem to exist for such men and women. And yet, they can have troubles of their own — they can be too skinny!

Clothing can help here and there and "upholster" some places a little, where natural upholstery is lacking. Remember, however, not only plump people look older but very thin people, too! Often their movements are angular and stiff — they lack grace and agility, as well as buoyancy.

It may sound like a paradox that exercise will make you slim and it will increase your weight. This really depends of course on your choice of exercises. Never think: "I don't need exercise. I'm too skinny, anyway!" It's not true. Where it is necessary for plump people to remove layers of fat by means of strenuous bodily movements, the exercises for thin people lean towards lighter movement and relaxation.

A few tips: People who are too thin often have a restless nature. Compel yourself to rest. Now and then, get a change of air. Eat plenty of calorie-rich foods. Instead of eating three heavy meals a day, break them up into a number of smaller meals, so you don't overburden your stomach at any one time. What is forbidden to all others is permitted to you. Eat moderate amounts of sweets between meals, if you wish.

Now for the exercise.

Exercise 8: Extend your right leg to the side, stretch it, and raise your arms upwards to the left; inhale. Then draw the right knee up high pointing it to the left. Swing your arms to the right; exhale. Repeat four times; then perform the same exercise with all movements on the opposite side.

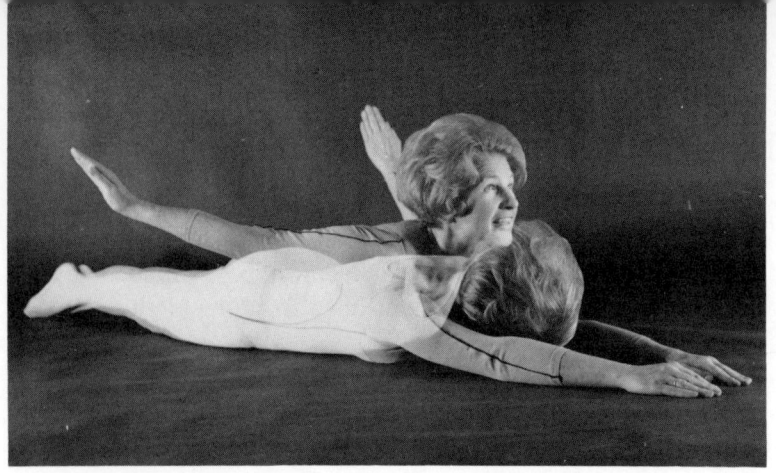

EXERCISE 9:
Start your daily routine by getting all the kinks out of your mind and body! Lie flat, face down, stretch legs back and arms forward as far as you can. Then lift your head and chest slowly and swing arms back slowly. Repeat four times.

DAILY EXERCISING

Whether you do your work seated or standing, there is a certain amount of physical exertion involved. Sitting motionless, standing for hours, running around — none is ideal for your well-being. Aching legs and feet, back pain, neck cramps, and a general feeling of weariness contribute in no way to enjoyment of your work. On the contrary, you count the hours and then collapse, grateful for just having managed to stagger through one more day. Why suffer this burden when you can do something about it? Get your body going. Prepare your muscles and joints for the exertion of work as well as your mind. You will find your work does not take as much out of you and you will not be worn out at the end of the day. Get more out of life, and enjoy the happiness and satisfaction that work brings to it.

Don't let even the tiniest trace of laziness in your make-up take over. You can forget about offering excuses, beginning with, "I-have-no-time," and continuing on to "I'm-too-tired," just to spare your body the imaginary "misery" of physical exertion. Just concentrate on the fact that besides contributing to good health and enjoyment of life, exercise also gives you that self-assurance which is absolutely necessary in the busy, pressured world we all live in today. Who has not experienced the pain and self-consciousness of awkward movements, from a nervously spilled coffee cup at a dinner party, to the agonizing paralysis brought on by a job interview? You are certain ahead of time you will do something wrong,

EXERCISE 10:
Lie on your back, and "pedal a bicycle." Every so often, without stopping the leg movements, sit up and exhale. Then slowly lie back down again, still pedalling.

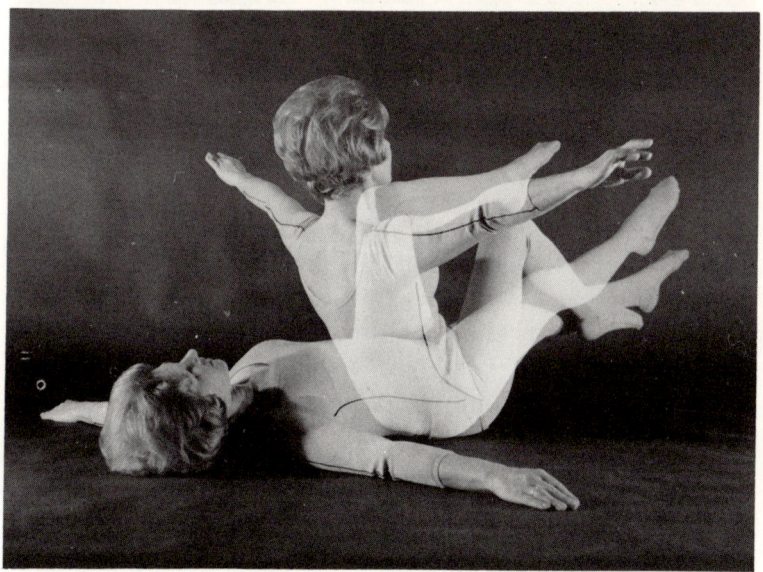

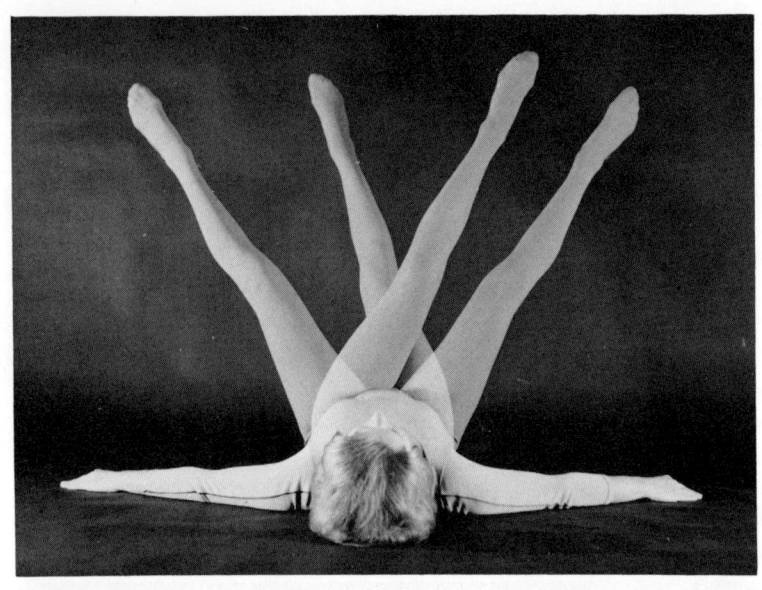

EXERCISE 11:
Lie flat on your back, arms spread wide, palms flat on floor. Raise your legs straight and open them wide. Then cross them — first left over right; then right over left.

that you will be inept and awkward. And you are right! However, a body conditioned by exercise always moves with harmony and, consequently, assurance.

Perhaps a little muscle-stiffness will hit you after your first attempt at exercising, just to show you how flabby and rusty your muscles and joints are! However, if you endure this mild punishment for neglecting your body, you will soon find yourself feeling better after each exercise session. Spend a quarter hour exercising each day and the exhaustion and unhappiness brought on by a tough work day will dissolve into thin air!

IF YOU SIT ALL DAY . . .

Actually, sitting forms a large part of all working conditions. Just think of the immense number of people with "sit-down" jobs, such as seamstresses, taxi drivers, computer operators, stenographers, even airline pilots! In all these jobs a person is virtually nailed down for hours on end to the same seat. It's not hard to understand how sitting leads to a pad of fat around the hips. However improbable it may sound: Too much sitting makes you not only flabby but tired! Posture is easily forgotten and as a result, breathing is impaired. Short-

EXERCISE 12:
Lie flat on your back, arms extended straight behind your head. Then swing yourself to a sitting position, at the same time raising one leg, and, bringing your arms forward, clap your hands under the raised leg, all the while exhaling. Lie back and inhale.

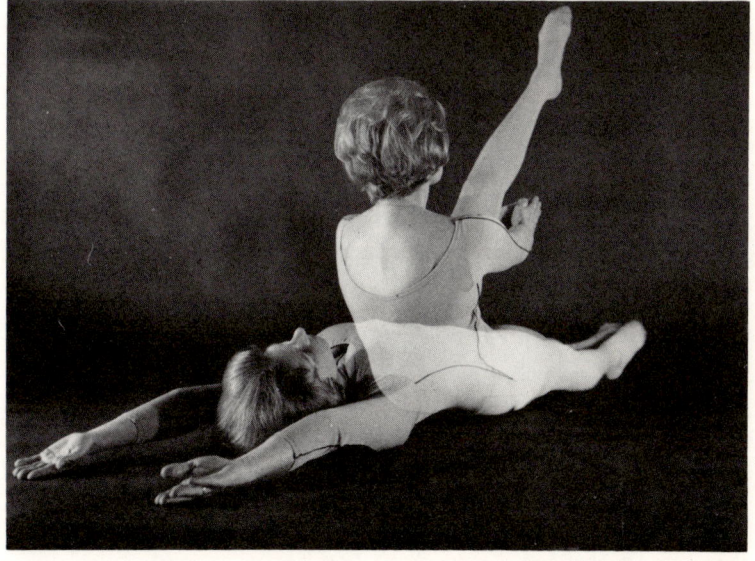

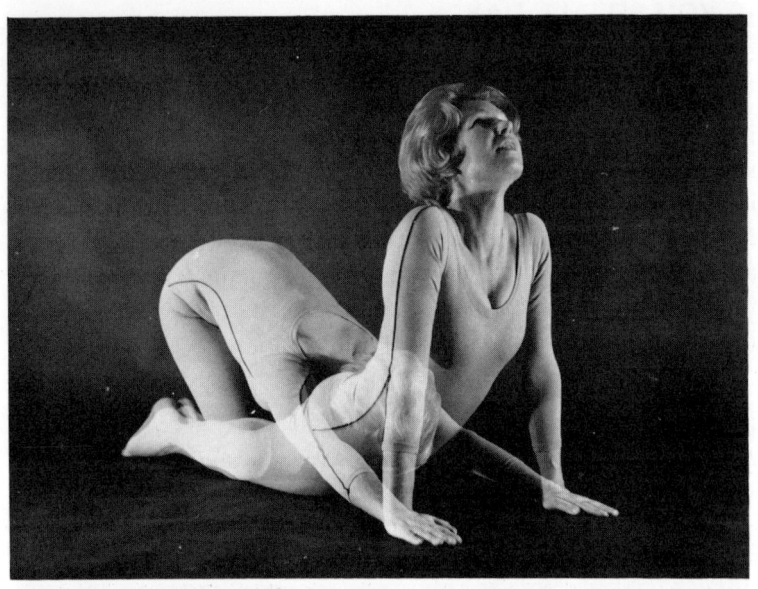

EXERCISE 13:
On your knees, head down, arms extended. Thrust your pelvis as far back as possible. Exhale. Then thrust your body forward, weight on your stiffened arms, head high, legs extended to the rear, and inhale.

ness of breath and poor circulation are the rule, not the exception. Therefore, if you have to sit a lot, stand up from time to time (you can always find some excuse for it), take a few quick steps to stimulate your body. Walk upstairs and back down again if this is possible; steal a couple of deep breaths of fresh air at an open window. Make sure your legs get a workout — remaining in one seated position with even the slight pressure of the chair edge against the underside of your thighs leads to poor circulation. Now, try Exercises 9 through 14 and see if you don't feel better immediately!

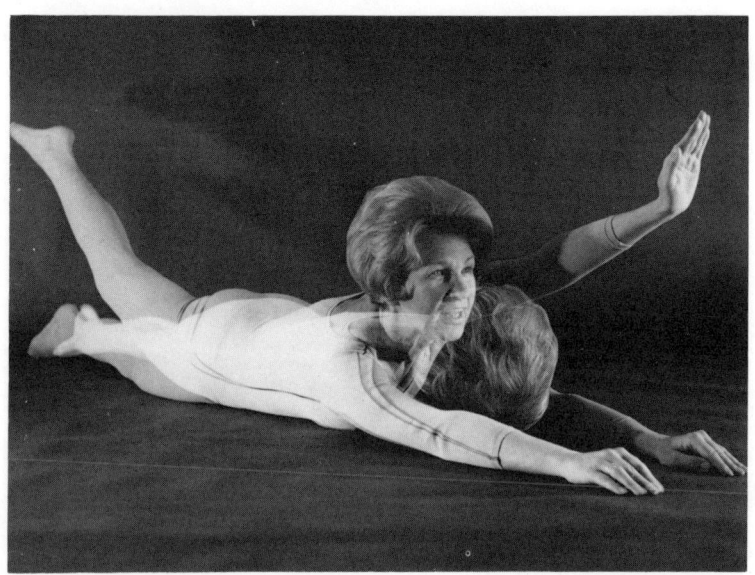

EXERCISE 14:
Lie flat on your stomach, and raise your right leg and left arm simultaneously; inhale. Drop back again. Exhale. Then raise your left leg and right arm.

IF YOU STAND ALL DAY . . .

Everyone, for one reason or another has had the experience of constant standing, such as on a bus or subway, or waiting in line at a bank on payday! So, imagine the physical strain on a teacher, a dentist, a waitress, a hairdresser, or a sales clerk!

If you are an all-day stander, or even an occasional one, your legs are overworked beyond their capacity! As soon as your feet begin to ache, you fall into a stooped posture,

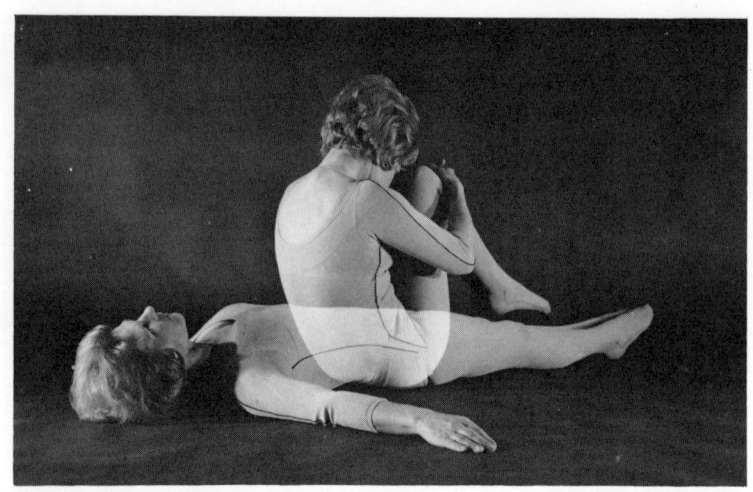

EXERCISE 15 (above)

EXERCISE 16 (below)

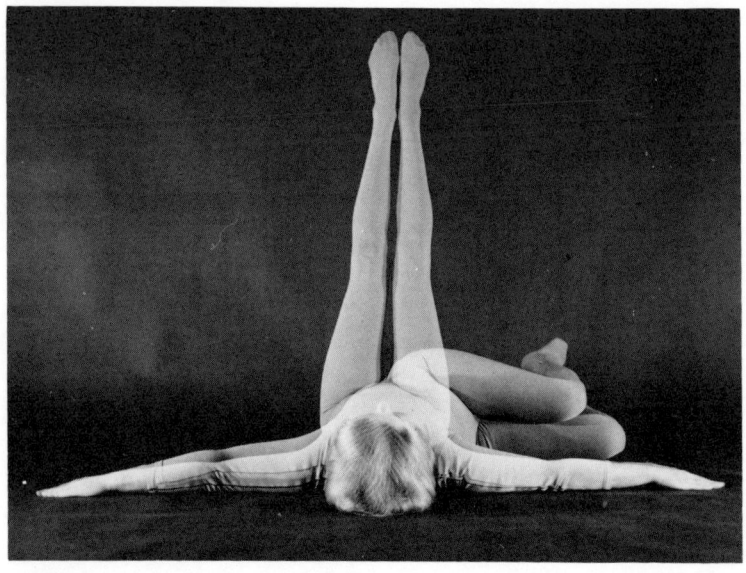

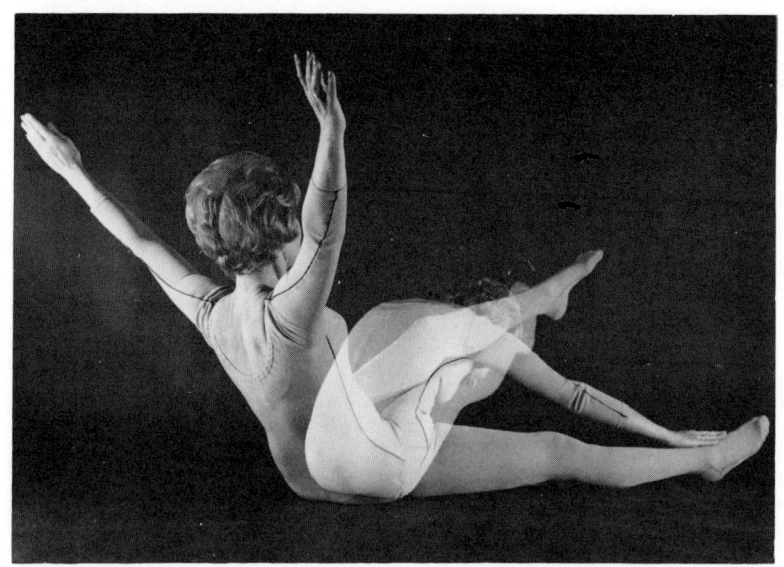

EXERCISE 17

EXERCISE 15:
Lie on your back. Sit up slowly, and bend both legs up towards you, clasping them with your arms. Exhale. As you lie back down, inhale.

EXERCISE 16:
Flat on your back, arms outstretched, palms pressed against the floor, bring your legs up, knees stiff. Exhale. Bend your legs, and bring them down to the floor on the right. Inhale.

EXERCISE 17:
In a sitting position, stretch both arms up and out. Cross your outstretched legs twice, right over left, then left over right. Inhale. Bend forward, returning your legs to the outstretched position, and touch your ankles. Exhale.

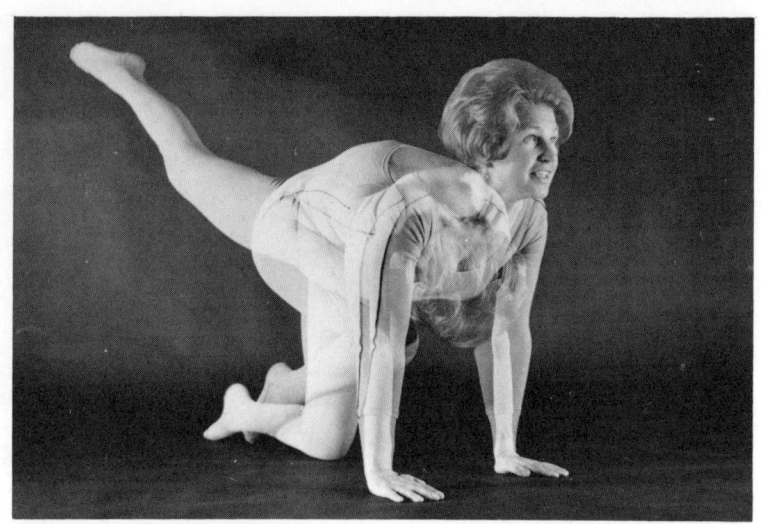

EXERCISE 18 (above)

EXERCISE 19 (below)

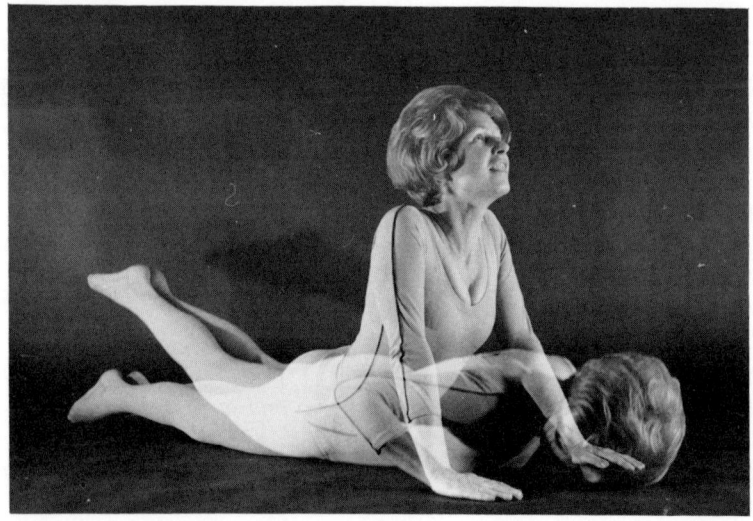

EXERCISE 18:
On your hands and knees, bend your head down. Draw one leg forward, knee towards your forehead. Round your back. Exhale. Then swing the leg back and up, stretching your back. Inhale. Repeat, using other leg.

EXERCISE 19:
Lie flat on floor, face down. Push your torso up by straightening and stiffening your arms, as if doing a push-up, hands supporting the body weight directly beneath the shoulders. Inhale. Slowly lower yourself down. Exhale.

your back becomes hollow, and you destroy your figure. Besides, who can be eager about work and have a friendly air, if plagued by tired feet? Also, supposing you like to bowl occasionally in the evening, or play handball, or even take a dip in a pool, how can you if you are just plain exhausted every day? If this applies to you, work on Exercises 15 through 19.

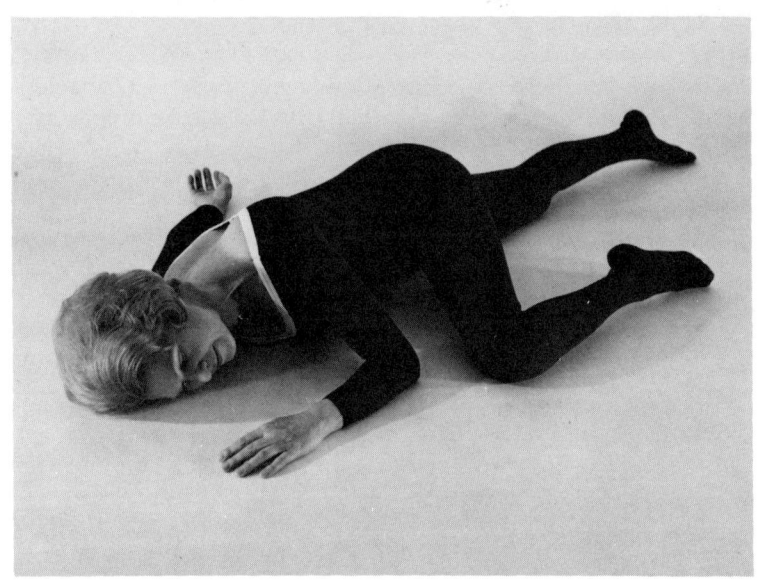

RELAXATION

Why relax? In the hurry and bustle of daily life and because of excessive demands that preparation for sports puts on your strength, you need complete relaxation at the proper time in order to be able to create new energy. Every long-lasting game or exertion leads necessarily to cramping up. Each cramping up takes away your desire to play, your pleasure, and prevents you from doing your best in sports.

When to relax? Don't wait until the game is over and you are overtired, to relax. Relax before the day of an important game, before tests, before guests arrive, before a visit to a theatre or concert. Then after a game, after periods of excitement and irritation, after periods of strain and success, you will be able to relax without being so overtired that you are tense.

What is the best way to relax? In a relaxed position! The photo shows you exactly how. Lie on your right side, because if you lie on your left side you will constrict your heart. Bend your left leg up and the right one out on the floor, so that your body is supported by the left knee. Rest your left arm in a bent position, so that your hand is opposite your face. Stretch your right arm out in the opposite direction, so that your right shoulder rests on the floor, and the palm of your hand faces up. Now close your eyes, let yourself "fall" (that is, make yourself feel heavy), and breathe deeply and slowly. The more fully and deeply you breathe, the more completely you relax! Think of waves on the sea, of a field of wheat undulating in the breeze. Better still, think of nothing! After a short time of complete relaxation, you will feel reborn!

This relaxed position is very definitely not an artificial position. Notice that it is this same position that newborn babies instinctively assume when they sleep. This is because it is the most completely comfortable sleeping position. Self-relaxation helps also to counter insomnia due to physical and nervous exhaustion.

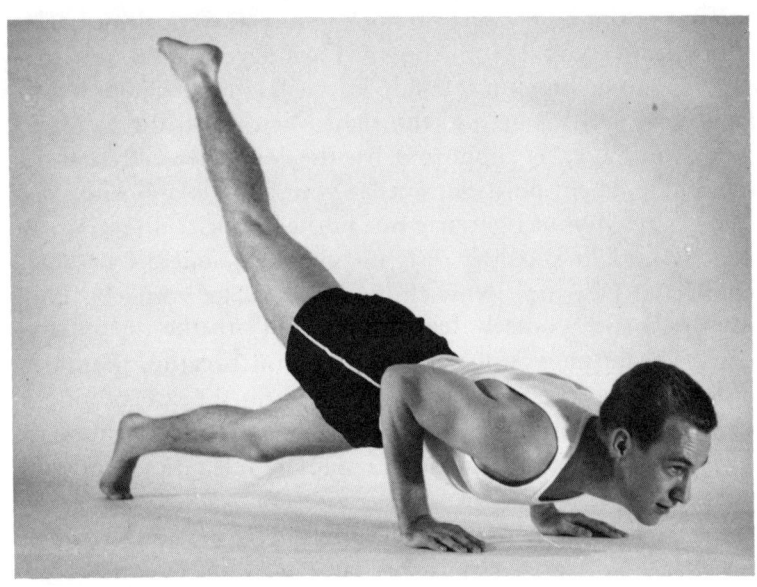

EXERCISE 20:
Make this simple test to see what condition you are in. If you can perform this exercise perfectly, you are in great shape! Assume a position where you are supporting your weight on your toes and hands with your arms straight. Slowly bend your arms, allowing your body to sink, at the same time lifting and stretching one leg. Exhale. Then repeat, lifting the other leg.

EXERCISES ESPECIALLY FOR THE SPORTSMAN

If your special sport is fishing or tennis or mountain climbing, here are a few tips that you can put to daily use at home, which will aid you greatly in general body-building. It takes only a little energy and a strong desire on your part to bring your physique back into line. You'll find that a few minutes of daily exercise will soon become a custom you simply cannot do without.

Exercise not only produces a good physique, but it brings

with it a feeling of well-being, renewed physical energy and creative energy which affect both your work and your private life.

And now a very important piece of advice for the entire family: Once a person has gotten to the point where he is willing to do exercises at home, don't tease him about it. Don't embarrass him if, at first, in doing a knee-bend, he has to grab hold of something or if his joints make creaking noises. Instead, join in and exercise with him. Remember, practice makes perfect.

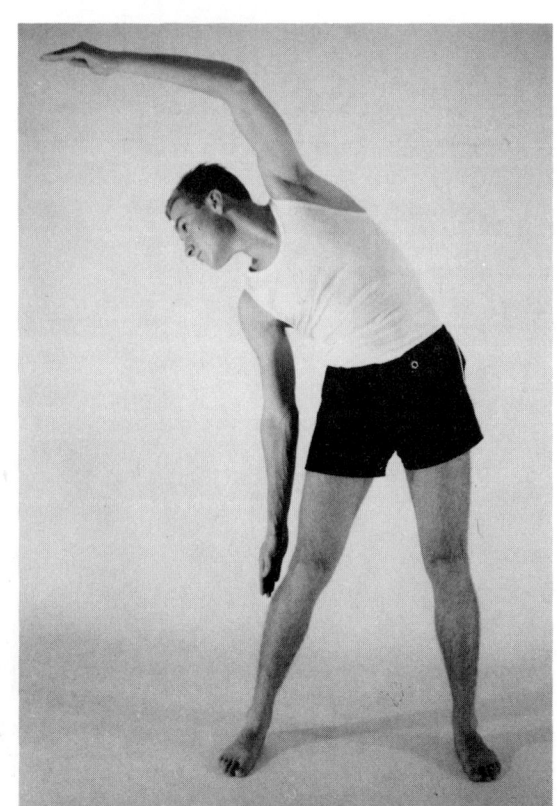

EXERCISE 21:
Getting started. Stand with feet apart and bend your torso twice far over to the right, straighten up, and then fall forward limply. Straighten up, bend twice to the left, and repeat. Inhale while doing the side bends; exhale while falling forward.

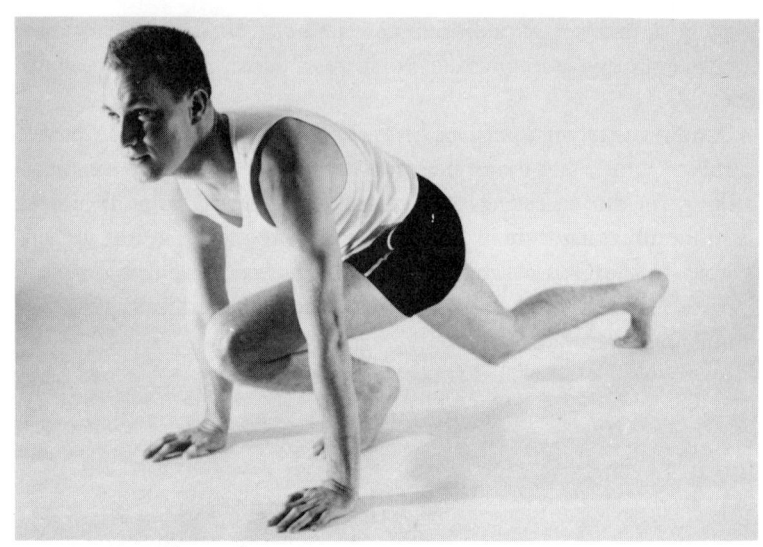

EXERCISE 22 (above)

EXERCISE 23 (below)

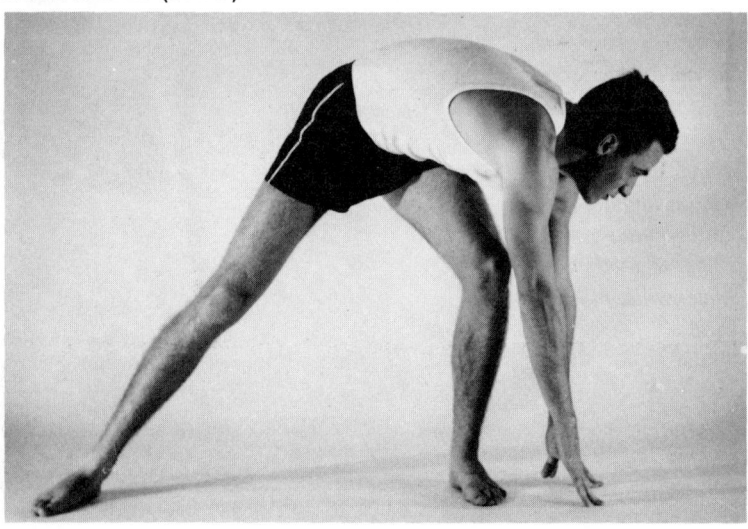

EXERCISE 24

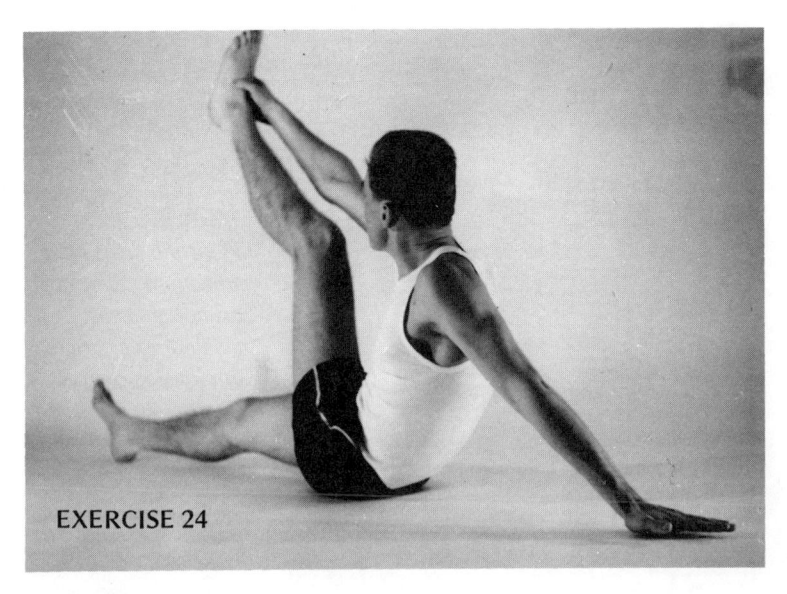

EXERCISE 22:
For your legs. Racing position, one leg stretched back, support yourself on bent leg and hands. Do two deep bends backward, bending your arms to lower your body. Then, quickly transfer the weight back to your arms and spring up, switching legs in the same position, so that the other leg is outstretched, and again do two deep bends.

EXERCISE 23:
For suppleness around the waist. Standing with feet wide apart, bend the weight of your body to the left while bending your left knee, and touch the floor on the outer side of your left foot. Exhale. Then straighten up fully, inhale, and immediately repeat the exercise towards the other side.

EXERCISE 24:
To counteract a rigid back. In a sitting position, bend your left leg, holding the foot with your right hand under the sole. Now stretch the leg up, exhaling, then return to the original position and inhale. Do this ten times with the left foot, then ten times with the right. Even try it with both at the same time.

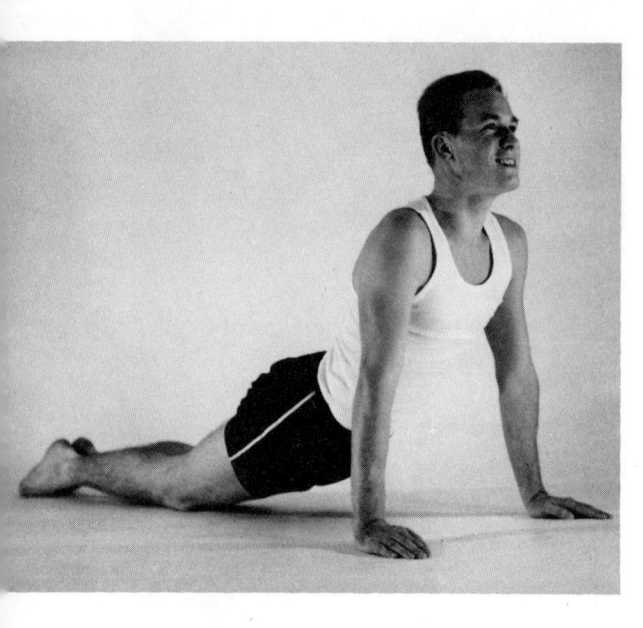

EXERCISE 25:
Lie prone, arms bent, hands under shoulders. Straighten arms, raising body. Inhale. Sink back slowly. Exhale. As you lift, try looking over your shoulder.

EXERCISE 26 *(below):*
Align your back properly. From an outstretched prone position, swing your arms backward and grasp your raised feet. Bow your body up. Inhale. Let go, drop back into the original prone position, and exhale.

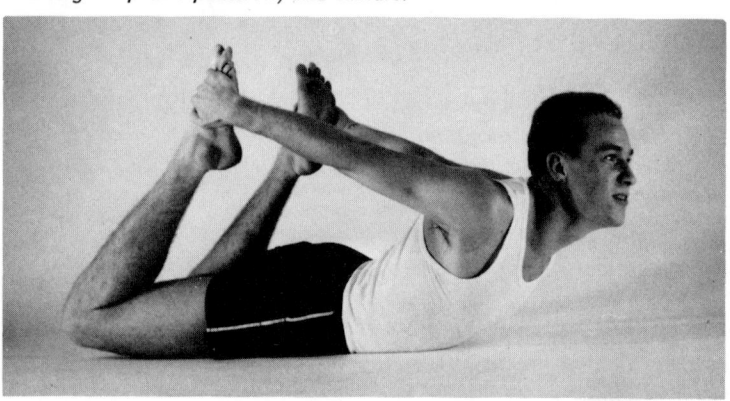

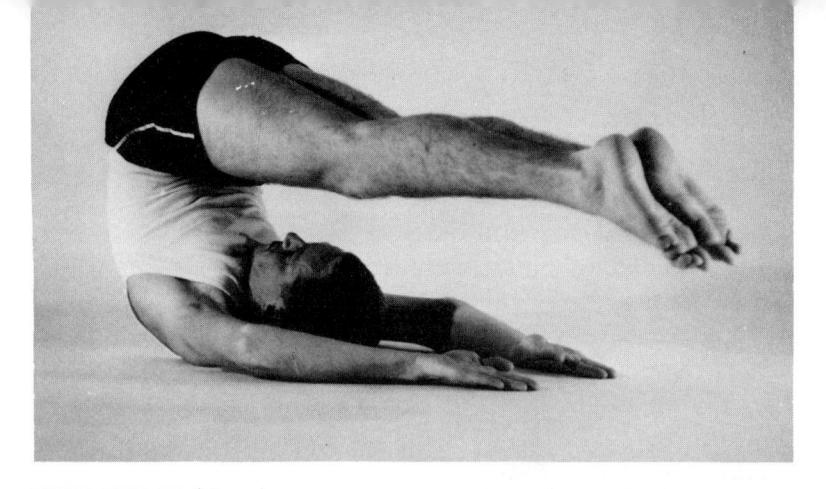

EXERCISE 27 *(above):*
From sitting position, roll over backward, swinging legs over head until toes touch floor. Exhale. Slowly return to sitting position, holding legs suspended. Inhale. Then bend forward, touch toes. Exhale.

EXERCISE 28:
Lying on shoulders, lift legs high and "bicycle." While "bicycling," slowly lower legs and rise to sitting position. Then lie back down, legs still moving, and raise them again to the original position.

BETTER POSTURE

Posture concerns two kinds of backbone: Your spinal column and your will to improve its condition! These pages are intended to put a halt to the all-too-common laziness that pervades easy-living societies. Unfortunately, during the school years, too little attention is paid to posture. Youngsters romp around and do all kinds of good natural activities to counteract the hours of sitting still at their desks, so body posture is less of a problem. But what was neglected then you must now make up for as soon as you can.

What has posture to do with sports? A great deal. If you are rigid, you can't hit the ball. On the other hand, your back muscles, so important to good posture, must be made elastic and strong.

The old military command: "Stick out your chest! Suck in your belly!" is definitely out! An erect posture does not come from a rigid "held-position" but from active movement. A slack posture is not only unattractive but it also prevents proper breathing. Whether you realize it or not, your posture reflects your attitude towards yourself. If you are unsure of yourself, it will show in the way you carry yourself. A few posture exercises, therefore, are a must in your exercise schedule. Get hold of a hand towel, an umbrella, or a yardstick — and get started!

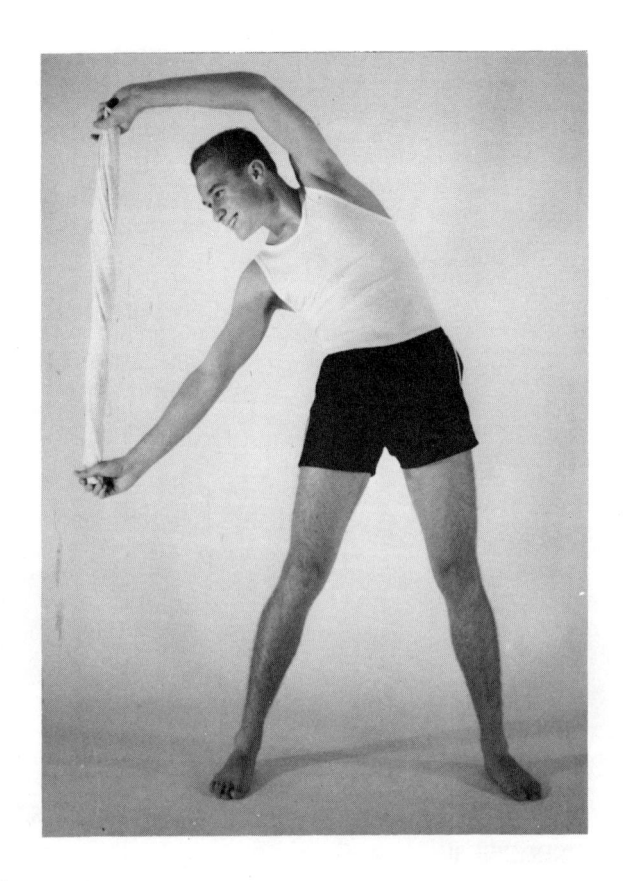

EXERCISE 29:
Standing with feet apart, swing your trunk in a circle. Stretch the towel between your two hands, bend over to the right, straighten up and inhale. Bend deeply to the left, and exhale. Then immediately swing over to the other side, the right side, and straighten up again.

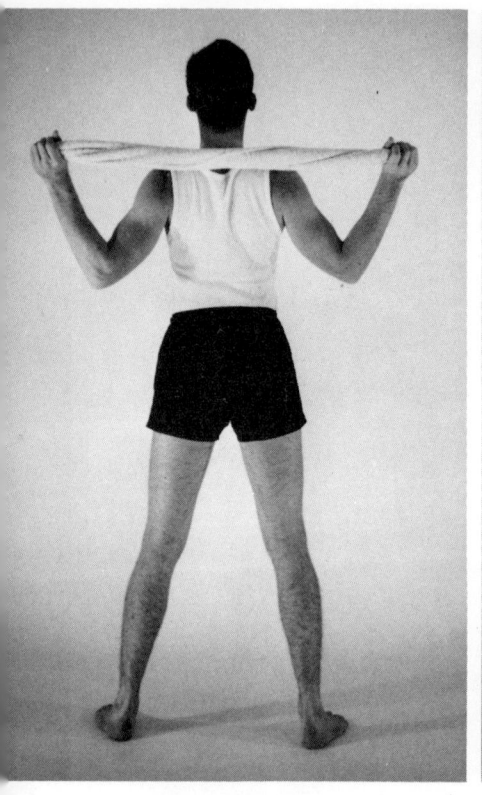

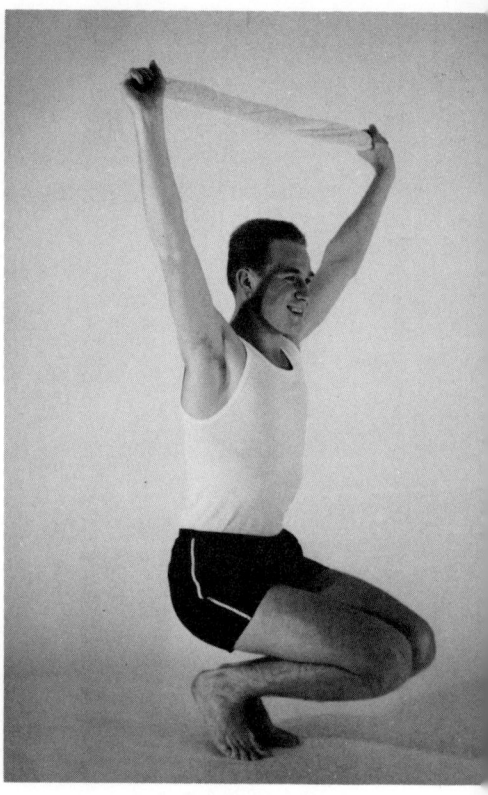

EXERCISE 30   EXERCISE 31

EXERCISE 30:
Standing erect, bring the towel across your shoulders, at the same time pushing your elbows backward, and inhale. Then stretch your arms up, bend your body forward, and exhale.

EXERCISE 31:
Legs together, arms at your sides. Quickly do a deep knee-bend, at the same time swinging your arms high and stretching the towel over your head. Inhale. Stand, drop your arms, and exhale.

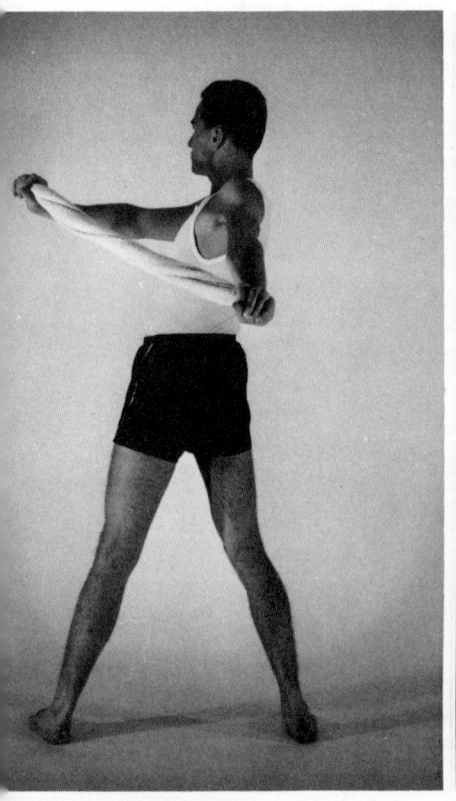

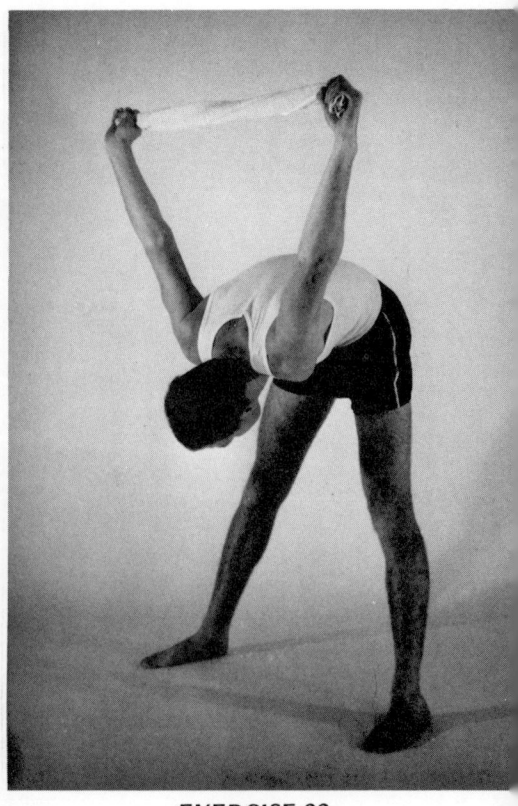

EXERCISE 32   **EXERCISE 33**

EXERCISE 32:
Feet apart, stretch the towel as far back to the left as possible. Do twice. Then repeat on the right. While turning, pull powerfully with your hands so that you spring back.

EXERCISE 33:
Feet apart, stretch the towel behind your thighs. Bend your body far forward, at the same time swinging your arms up. Bend back and exhale. Straighten up, bend your head back, and inhale.

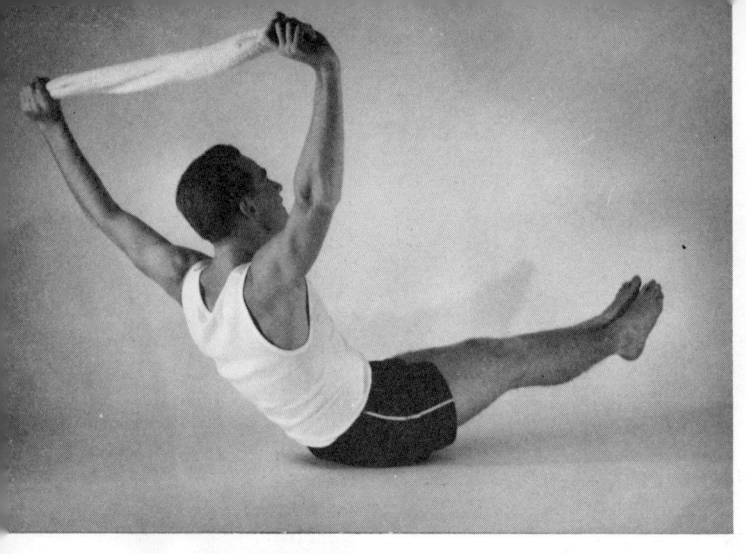

EXERCISE 34

EXERCISE 34:
Sit, legs stretched out. Drop the towel in front of your feet, and exhale. Swing your arms high over your head, at the same time raising your legs and stretching out. Inhale.

EXERCISE 35:
On your knees, body erect. Bend back and touch the floor behind your feet with your right hand. Exhale. Straighten up, relax, and inhale. On the next backward bend, turn to the left.

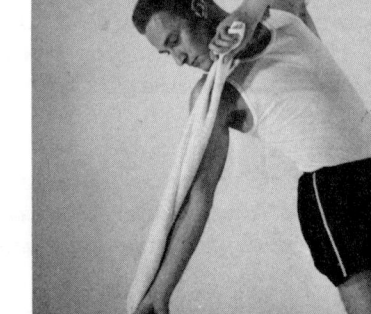

EXERCISE 35

EXERCISE 36:
Let your body hang forward. Swing once to the left; then once to the right. On the right swing, strain your right hand upwards. Then return and strain with your left hand.

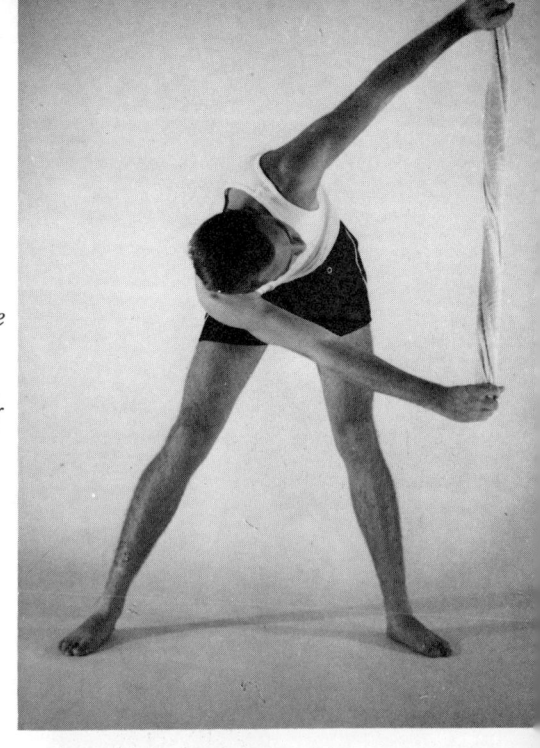

EXERCISE 37:
On your stomach. Raise the towel high. Lift your legs off the floor. Inhale. Hold this position of high tension for a short time; then sink back to a flat position, and exhale.

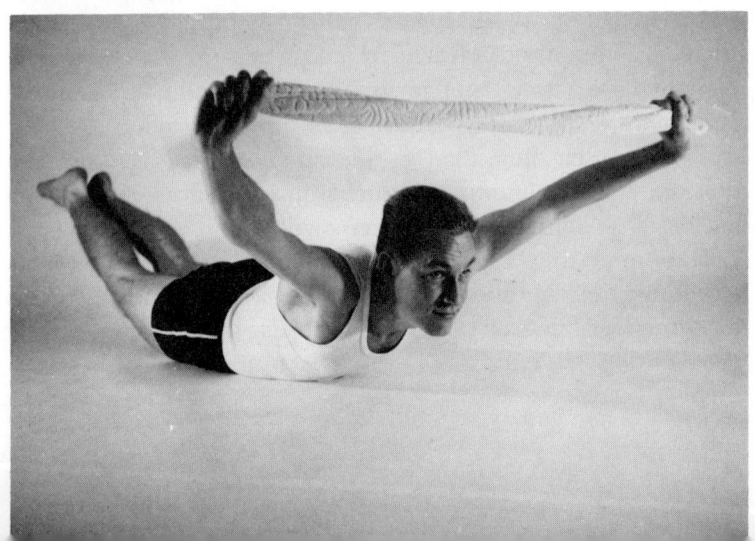

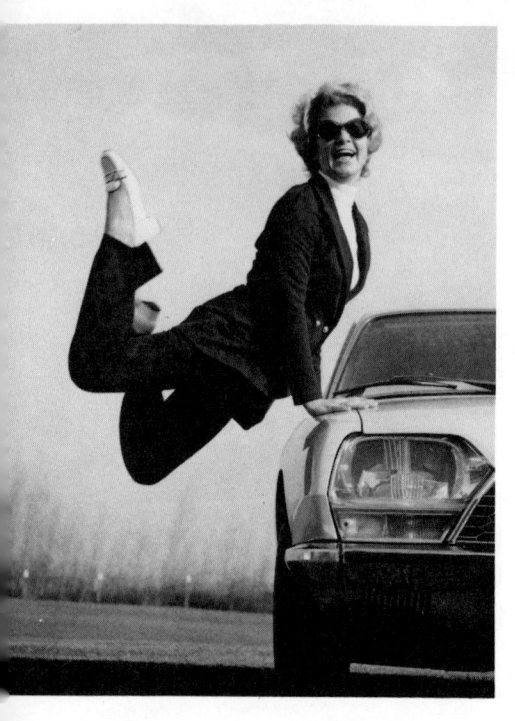

EXERCISE 38:
Take a few running steps, support yourself as shown and kick both heels upward behind you. Then spring away energetically.

TANK UP ON FRESH AIR

If you have to drive to your ski lodge, or golf course, or tennis court, or to the beach, you probably give your four-wheeled companion better care and attention than yourself! As you drive along, you probably don't make the slightest movement toward compensating or animating your muscles. Is it any wonder, then, that by the time you arrive at your destination you are cramped, your stomach tightened up, your back stiff or aching and your legs swollen?

How much better, in the interest of your health as well as travelling safety, now and again to make a brief stop! "Stretching your legs" is the old term for this, but limbering up is

EXERCISE 39:
Begin this series with an intensive breathing and stretching exercise! Swing your arms up and down vigorously twice. Inhale. Then let your trunk relax and fall forward. Exhale.

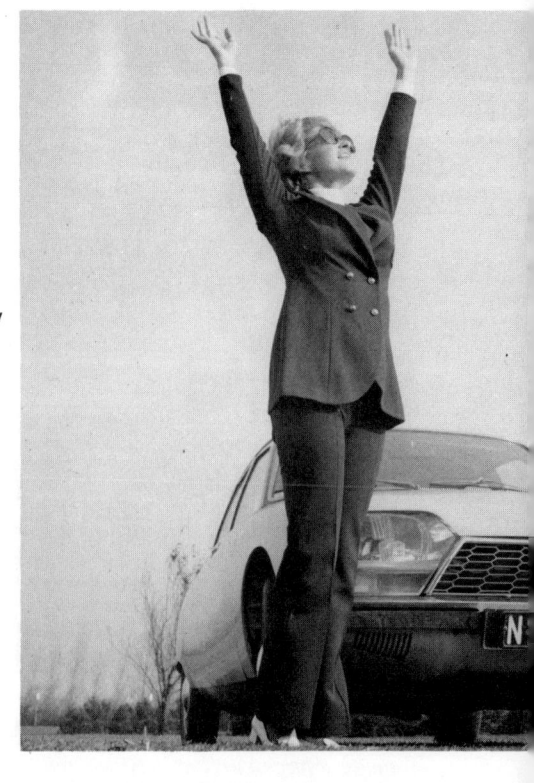

more like it. If you are with agreeable companions, you can make a game of these pauses. Take turns hopping up on the fender of your car as in Exercise 38. Strong coffee and raucous music may keep you alert in some circumstances, but frequent halts with short exercises will help you arrive at your destination feeling better. You will never be "broken on the wheel" if you try Exercises 39-43 when you stop driving — or travelling along as a passenger. It is not the driving or the kind of seat and springs that fatigues you — it is much more the lack of bodily movement.

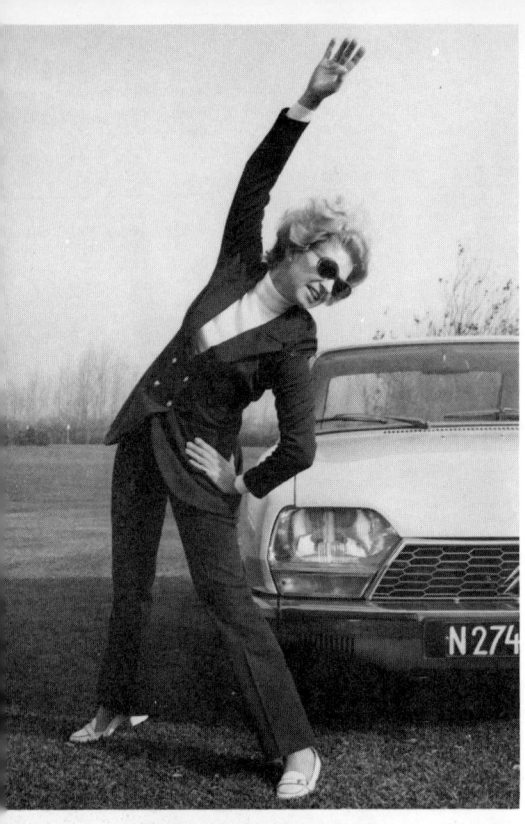

EXERCISE 40

EXERCISE 40:
For an elastic waist. Legs apart, left hand on hip, with your right arm make a large curve over your head to the left. At the same time, bend your torso deeply to the left. Exhale. Straighten up, and inhale. Quickly perform the same exercise towards the other side.

EXERCISE 41:
Stimulates circulation. First with the right leg, then with the left, make a wide, circular swing over the top of the radiator or over the trunk. Also, as you lift a leg, spring away.

EXERCISE 42:
Limbering your hips. Supporting yourself with both hands on the car, at the same time stretch one leg out behind you and swing it high. Exhale. Bring your legs together again, straighten up, and inhale. Repeat with the other leg.

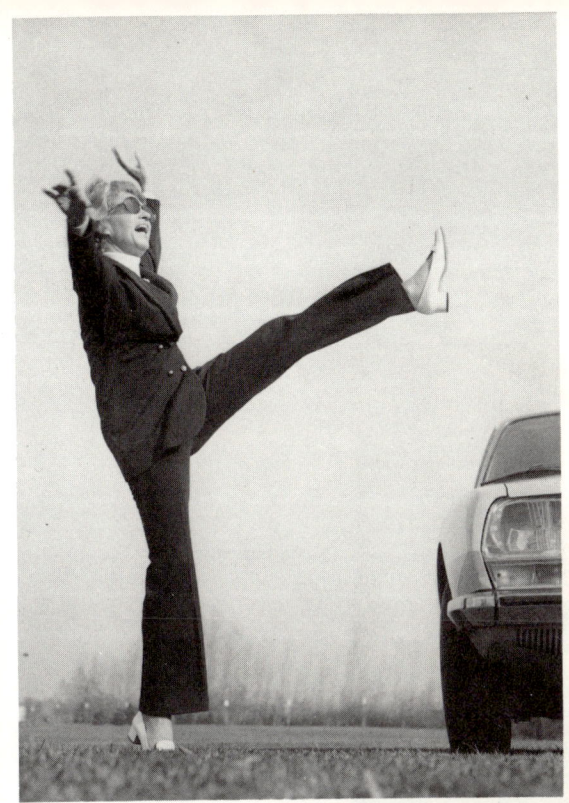

EXERCISE 41

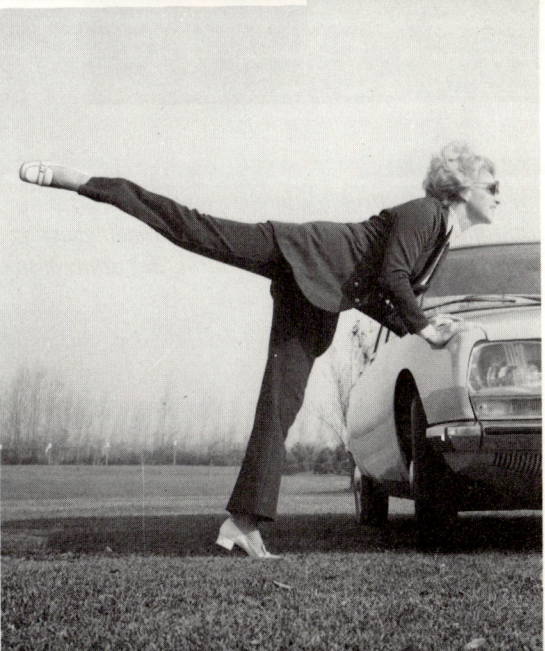

EXERCISE 42

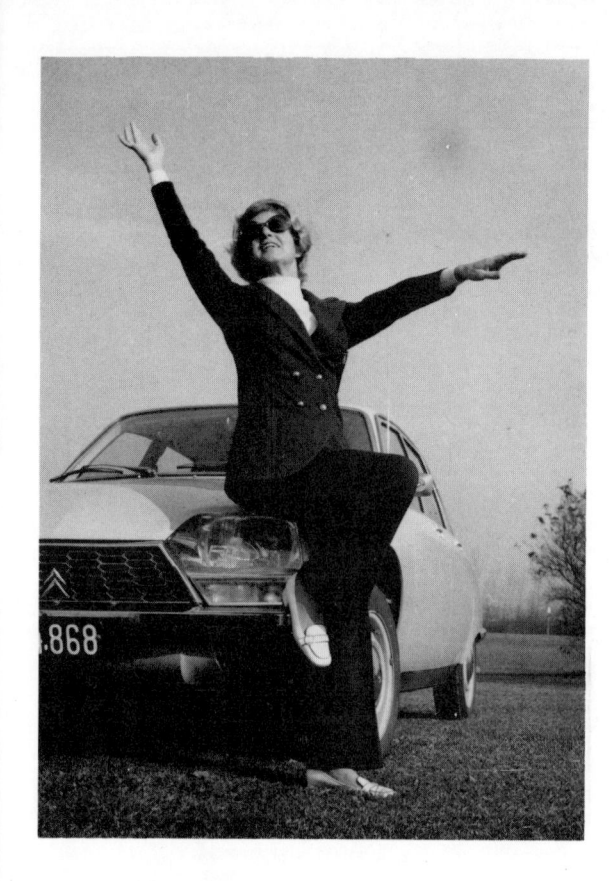

EXERCISE 43

EXERCISE 43:
For posture. Stretch your left arm out in front of you, and your right arm up high. Push the raised arm straight back at the shoulder twice. Then change arm positions, raising the other arm and pushing it back twice.

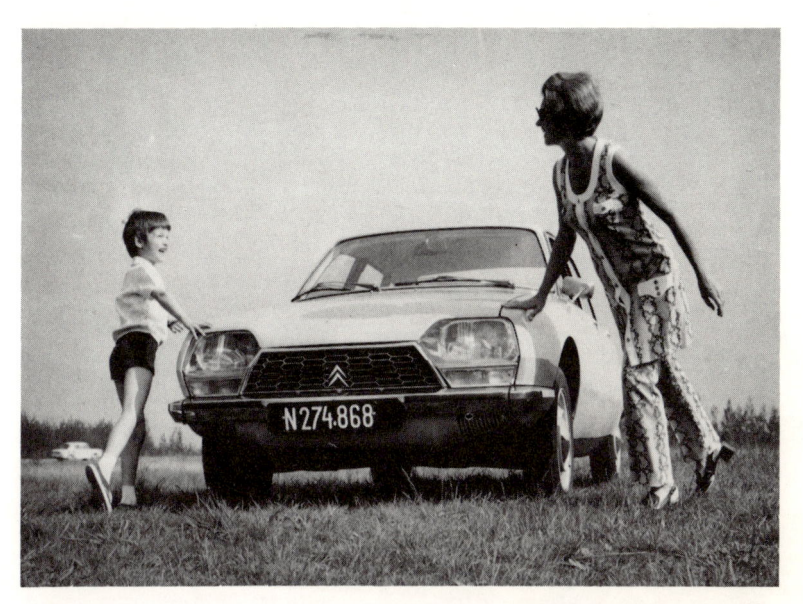

A GAME:
Catch me! Games of catch and races around the car from time to time will turn your outing into a really pleasurable event.

TRAVELLING WITH CHILDREN

How pleasant it is to be able to load the family, bag and baggage, into the car for weekend excursions and long vacation trips. It is hard enough for adults to have to sit still for hours on end, but it is even worse for children! No matter how anxious the little ones are to ride along in the car, they just as quickly tire of it, become restless and disturb the driver. Instead of enjoying the ride, you hurry along to arrive at your destination as soon as possible, with everyone getting crankier by the minute. But why not turn the trip itself into a game! Without warning, make a short stop to let everyone out and run around. As soon as you come to a field by the road make

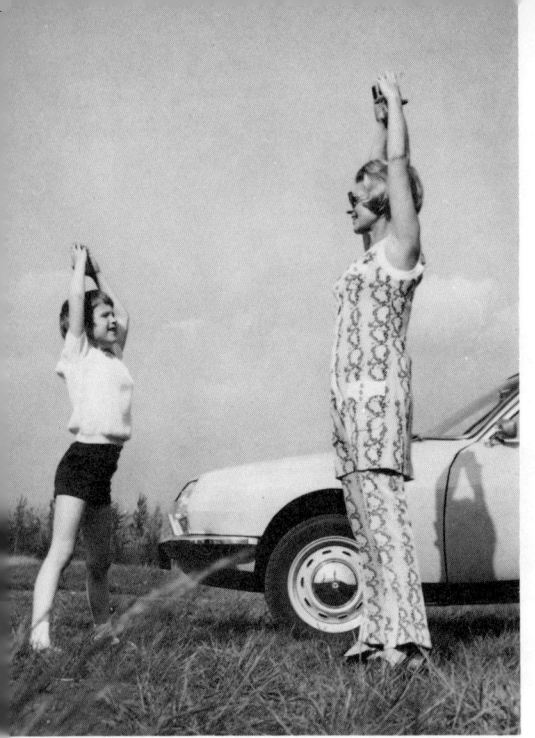

EXERCISE 44:
Do this, do that! Raise both arms above your head, then bend forward as far as you can. Swing your arms between your legs and exhale.

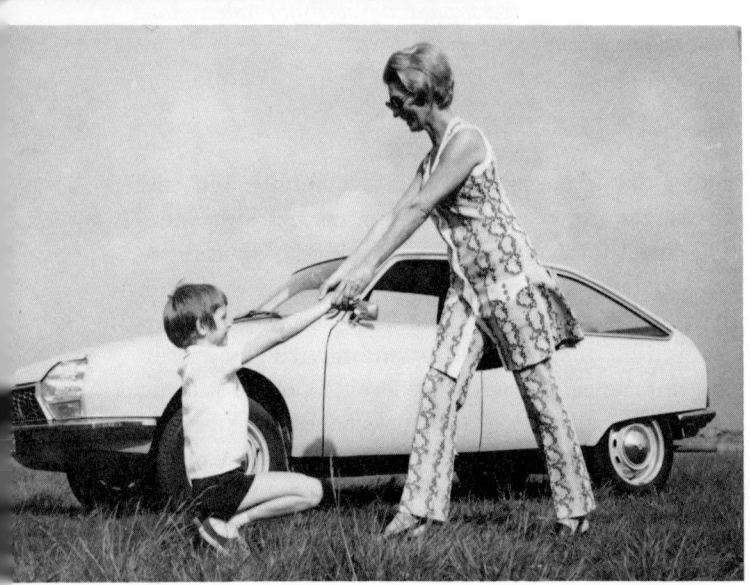

EXERCISE 45

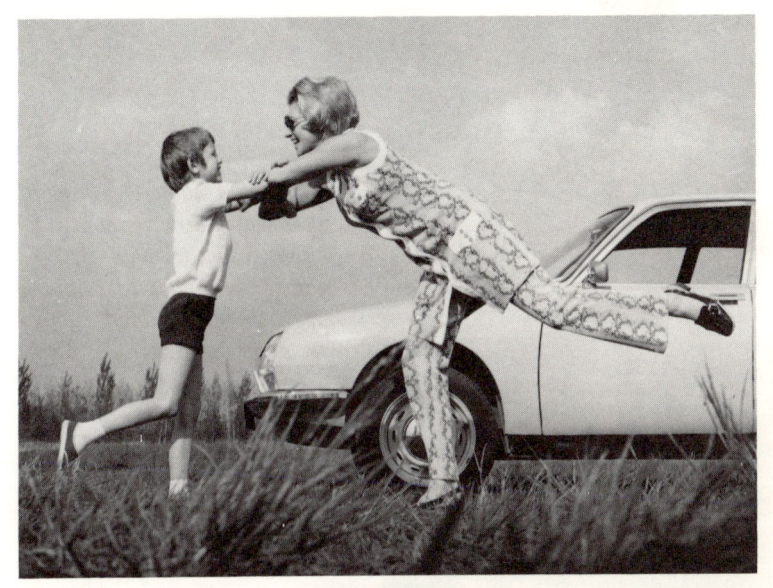

EXERCISE 46

a "fun and games" stop. Play catch or tag, turn somersaults, or stage a race — all these will make everybody happy and restore spirits. Tempers, as well as appetites, are sure to improve and everyone will look forward to the next leg of the journey. Besides, these exercises will stand you in good stead when you reach your destination. You'll be in better shape to swim, golf, or play any sport.

EXERCISE 45:
Round the Mulberry Bush! Bend your knees and squat way down, holding on to your partner with both hands. Then hop around in a circle like a bunny! Both children and adults.

EXERCISE 46:
One-leg Joust! Hop on one leg, with arms folded. Try to push your opponent off balance. Which one can stay longest on one leg? Then hop on the other leg.

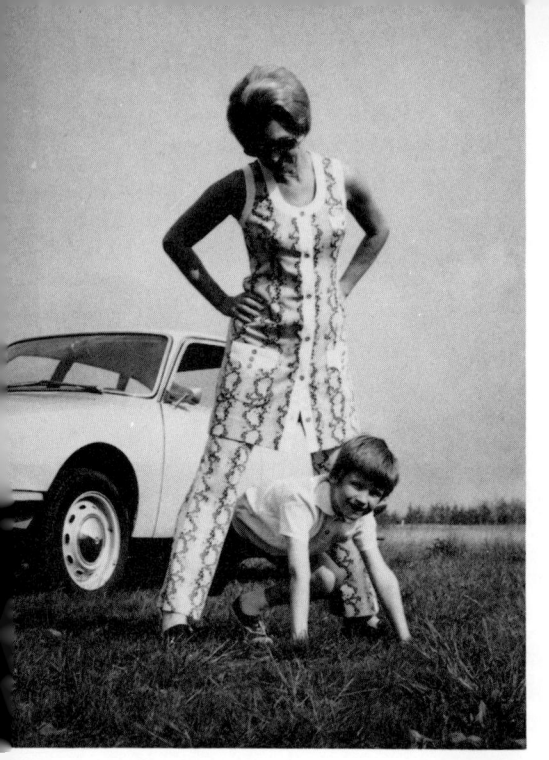

EXERCISE 47:
Through the Tunnel! An adult stands with feet apart and the children crawl through the "tunnel," run quickly around, and crawl back through again. Who is the fastest?

EXERCISE 48:
Tug of War! One person holds one leg thrust behind and the other holds it by the ankle. As one tries to hop forward, the other pulls back. Who is stronger? Every now and again, change legs and hop on the other one.

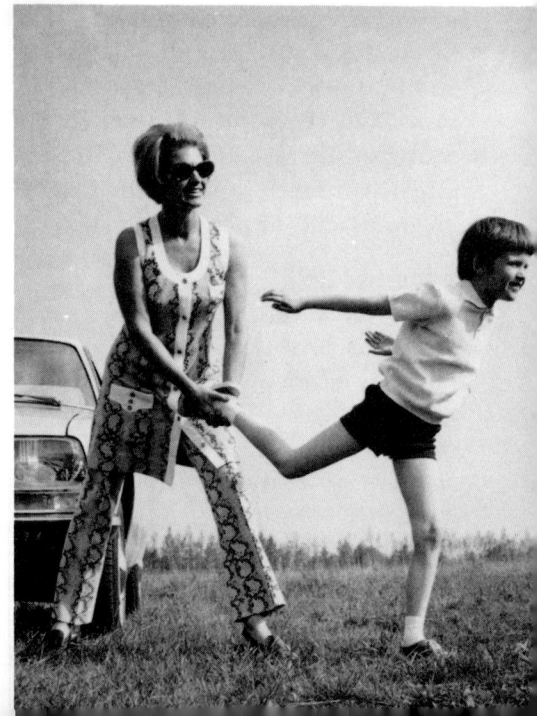

EXERCISE 49:
"Swinging" at home. With legs together, knees bent, press both heels forward, without raising them off the floor, first to the left, then to the right, swinging your knees loosely and swinging your arms in the opposite direction.

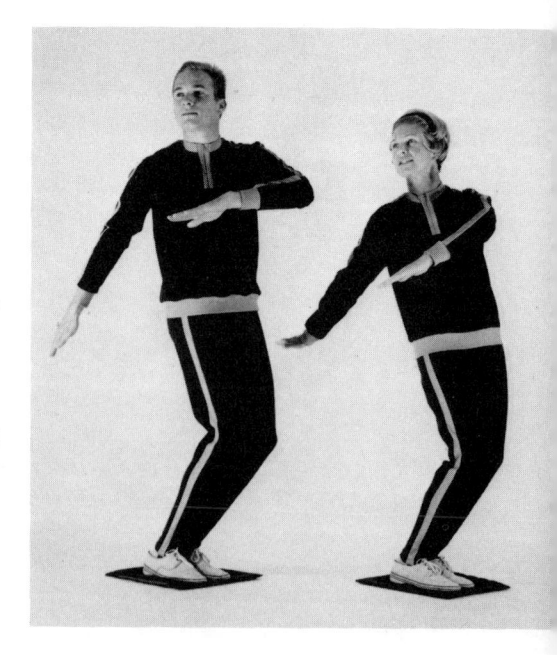

CONDITIONING FOR THE SLOPES

Is the skiing season coming up? Are you following excitedly the latest news from the snow country? Have you gotten all your equipment in shape? Well, whether you are an expert or a snow bunny, it is high time to get yourself into shape through proper conditioning and exercise. It would be a pity if a wrenched knee or stiff back on the first day out ruined your expensive weekend or vacation. And, just in case you decide at the last minute to head South for a golf vacation, remember — almost the same muscle movements are made in golf as in skiing, so all will not be lost!

The most important thing is to train for general body con-

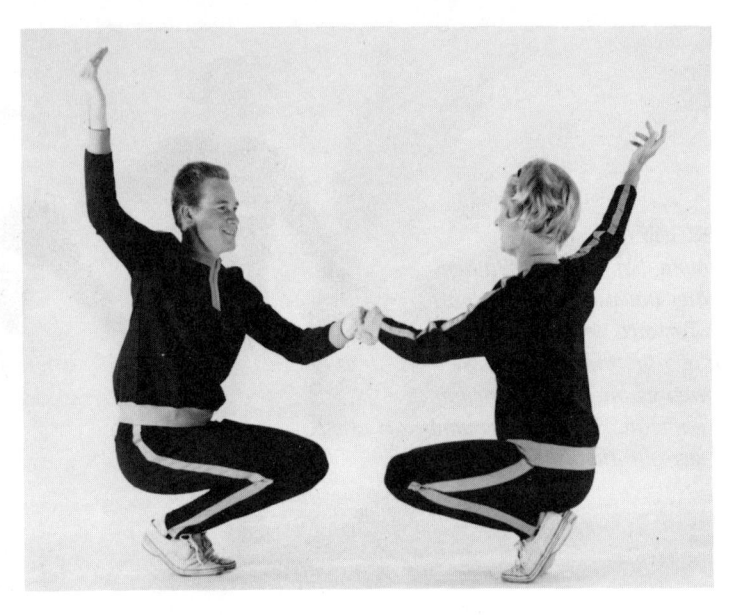

EXERCISE 50:
Grasp each other's left hands, and drop quickly into a deep knee-bend. Then pull each other erect. Repeat four times, then try it with the other hand.

trol and the ability to react, to strengthen your legs (especially to make the knee and ankle joints flexible) and not least, to prepare for general co-ordination and for confidence in speed.

Never has skiing been so full of dynamics as it is today. Never before has the harmony of technical ability and elegant movement been so complete as it is now. The "vacation skier," which includes most of us, has hardly any opportunity

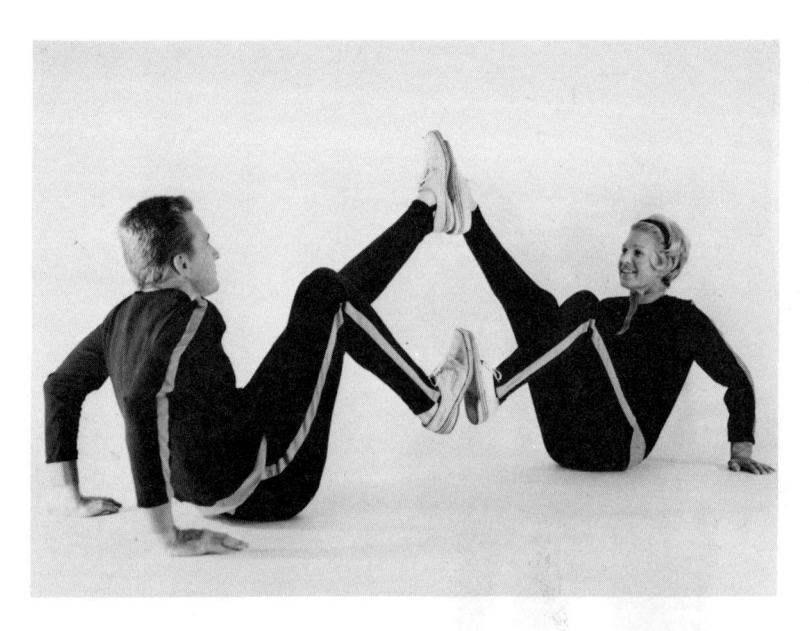

EXERCISE 51:
Sit opposite each other, supporting yourself with your hands, the soles of the feet pressed together and "bicycle." Push against each other's feet as you do it.

for actual conditioning training. The holidays and weekends providing snow are too few and far between to be ruined because you're not in shape. Even though you might spend the whole year industriously drilling away at various exercises, you will find the exercises on these pages will pay off when you hit the slopes that first day. Try them with a partner — it's even more fun.

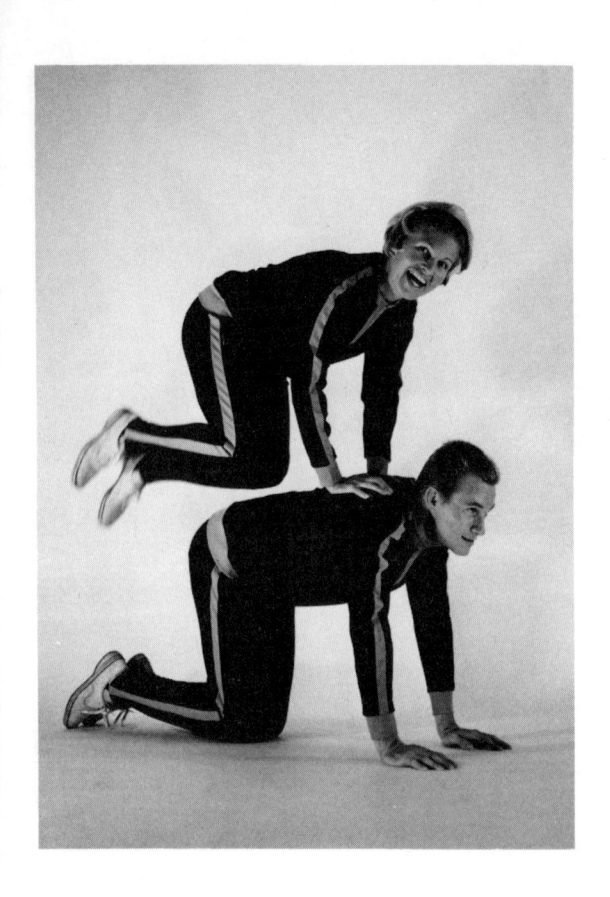

EXERCISE 52:

Leap-frog sideways over your kneeling partner! Rest your hands on his shoulder blades and stand beside him. Quickly, up with both legs, kicking your heels high up behind you, and land on the other side of him. After two brief, in-between hops, spring back the other way again.

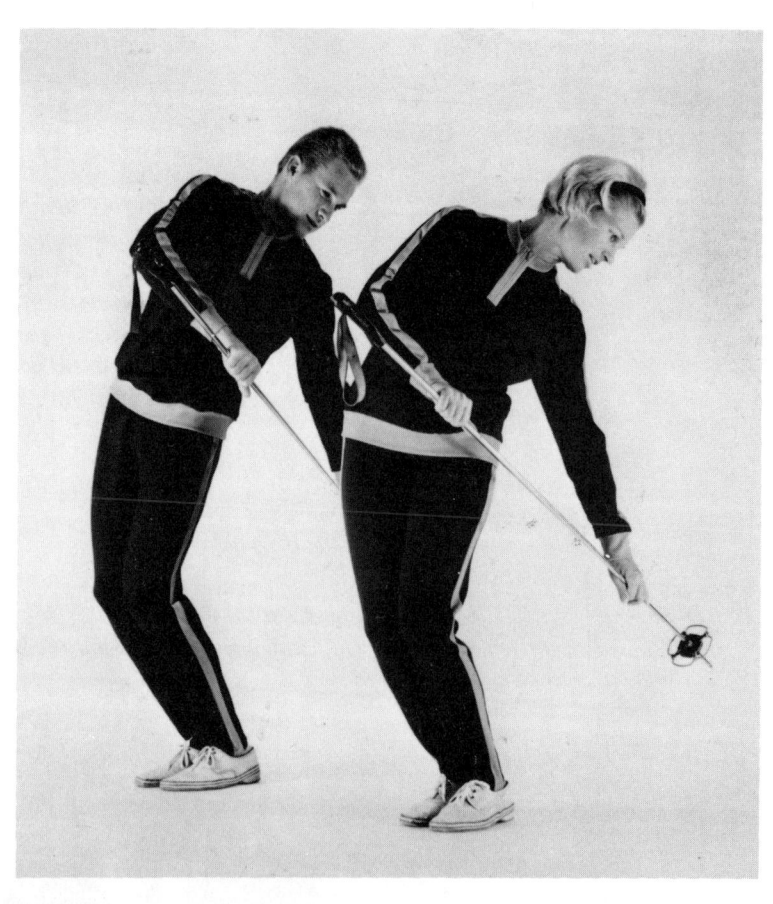

EXERCISE 53:
Hold the ski pole crosswise. Stretch one leg forward, sink slowly into a knee-bend, then pull yourself erect again. Repeat four times, then exercise again, standing on the other leg.

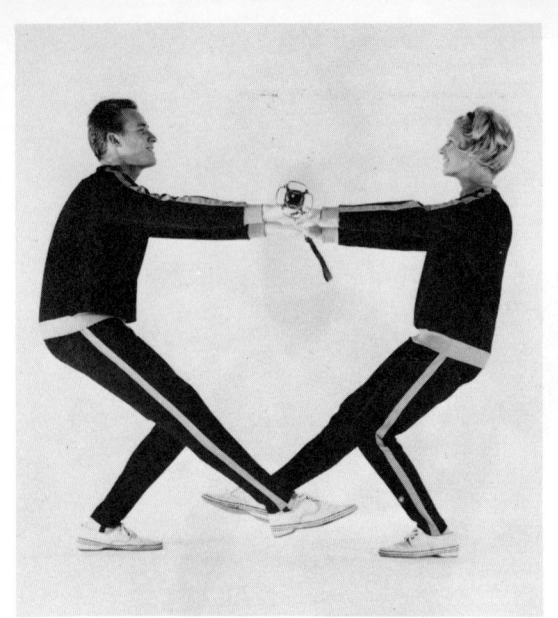

EXERCISE 54:
With legs together, hold a ski pole horizontally between you and your partner. Turn to the left and bend far over twice. Then straighten up and do the same to the right.

EXERCISE 55 *(below):*
Extend your left leg sideways over the ski pole. Bend sideways twice on your right leg. Then quickly straighten, and extend the other leg and again make two downward swings.

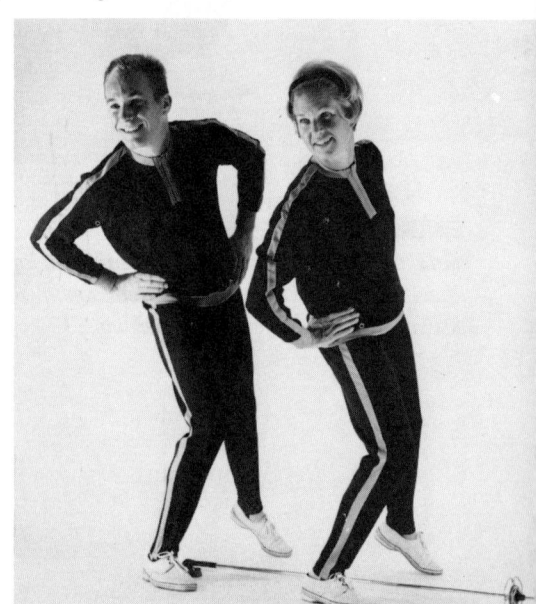

EXERCISE 55

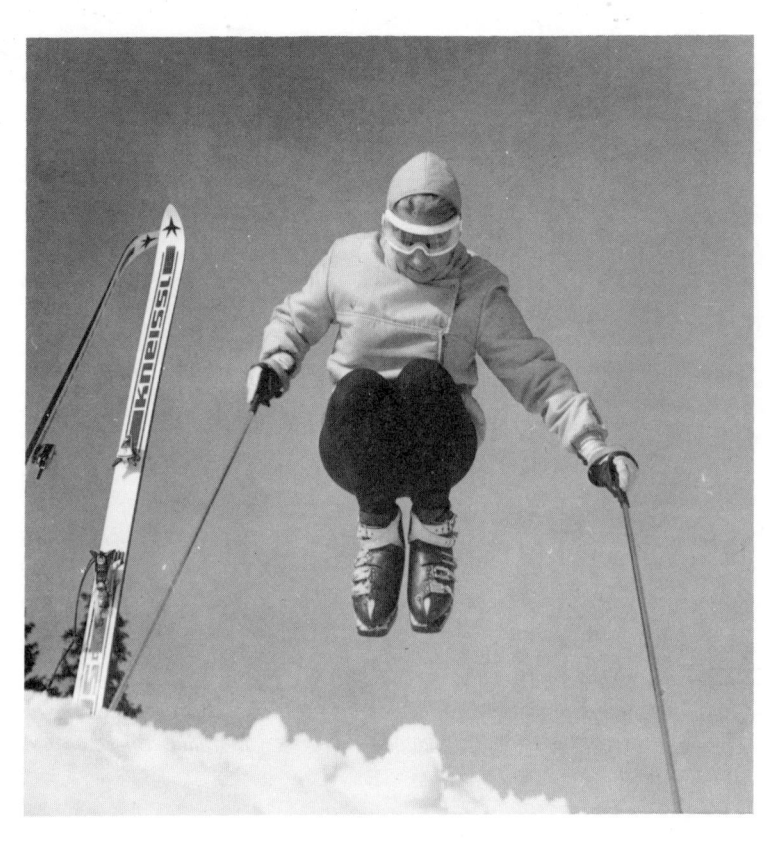

EXERCISE 56:
Supported on both ski poles, spring upward and pull your legs up high — a good exercise preceding the ski jump. Perhaps you can even turn left or right in mid-jump, or turn completely around.

PRACTICE ON THE SNOW

At long last, the skiing holidays are here. Everything is just as you want it: the weather is beautiful, you have done your at-home limbering-up exercises, you are in the best of moods,

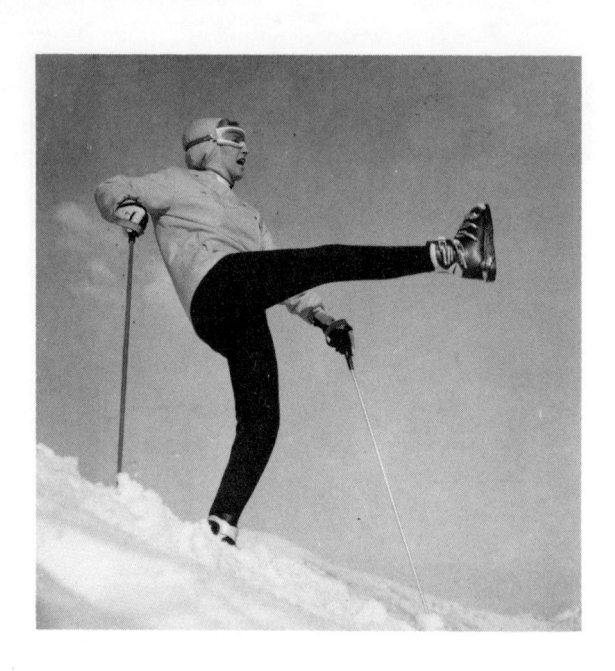

EXERCISE 57:
Supporting yourself on both poles, swing first one leg high in front of you, then the other. Your heavy ski boots will make this exercise appreciably more difficult.

and the companionship is perfect. But why are you standing up there on the track stiff and shivering with cold? Do you expect to push off in this condition? Before you buckle on your skis, or after a long trip on the ski-lift, you should go through some vigorous movements to warm up your blood.

Again and again you will observe beginners (otherwise known as snow bunnies) stand for a long time, getting stiffer and stiffer, and then suddenly, in this condition, not in full control, start the push-off. No wonder they often get dis-

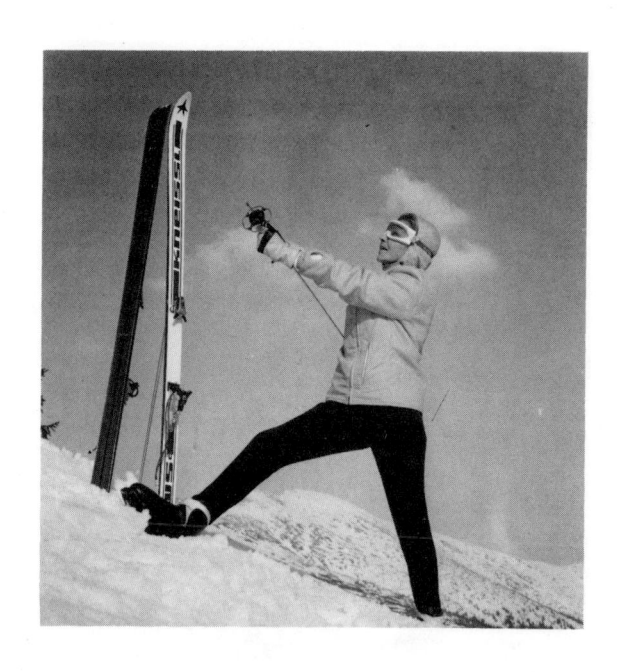

EXERCISE 58:
Stand with feet apart and swing a ski pole back to left and then to right, turning your trunk with the swing. Inhale. Then bend deeply forward towards the ground twice. Exhale.

couraged when they take header after header into the snow! If you are in class, while the instructor is explaining or the other students are practicing, try a few special exercises. In many children's ski classes, they do exercises over and over in between times. It's not only fun but it pays off in the form of greater progress.

The causes of most skiing accidents are "cold," or lack of good blood circulation in the muscles, and stiff joints. Suddenly, you have a strained ligament or a torn muscle. Whether

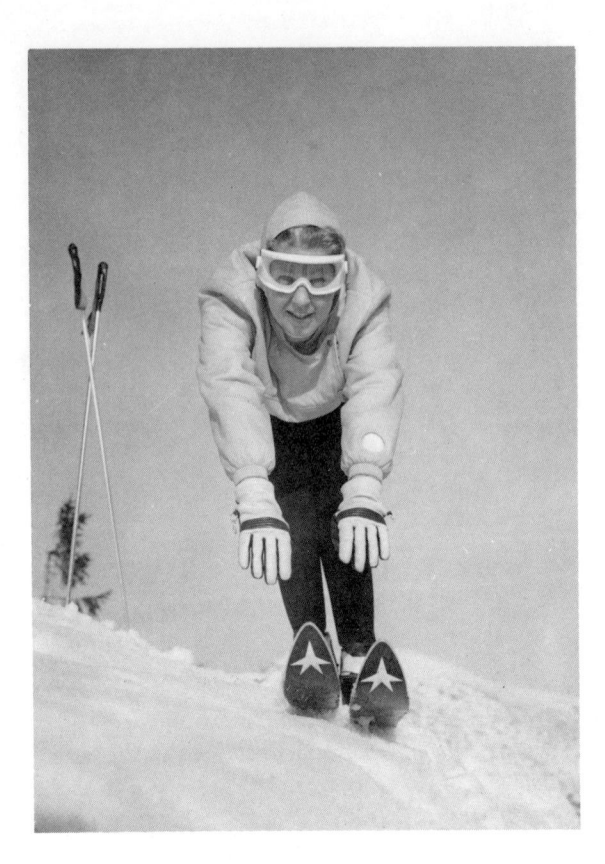

EXERCISE 59:
With skis on, bend your body far forward and take the weight off your heels, so the weight of your body falls on your toes. In this position, swing deeply from side to side a few times, then straighten up again.

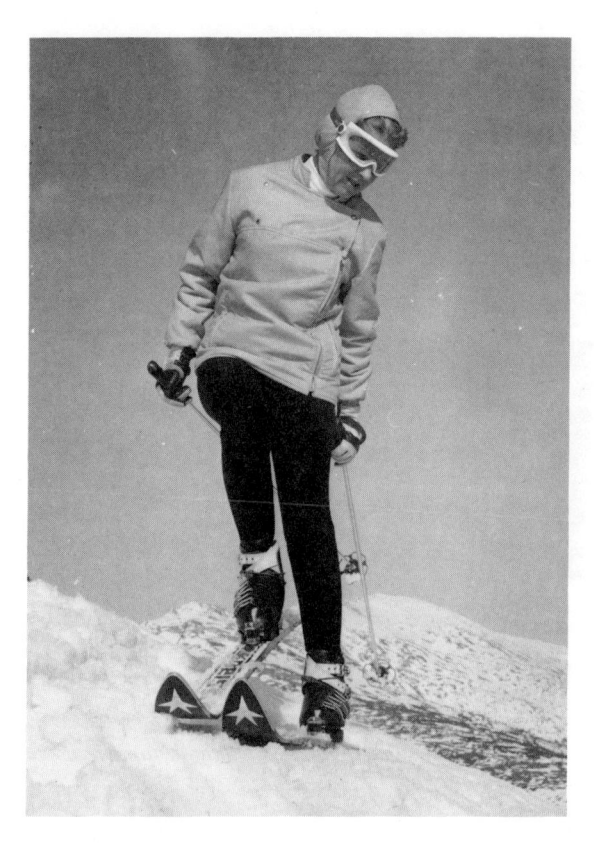

EXERCISE 60:
Put your weight on one leg. Vigorously lift first one leg and then the other, making sure to raise both ends of the ski off the ground. Do not keep the standing leg stiff, but flex it a little at the knee.

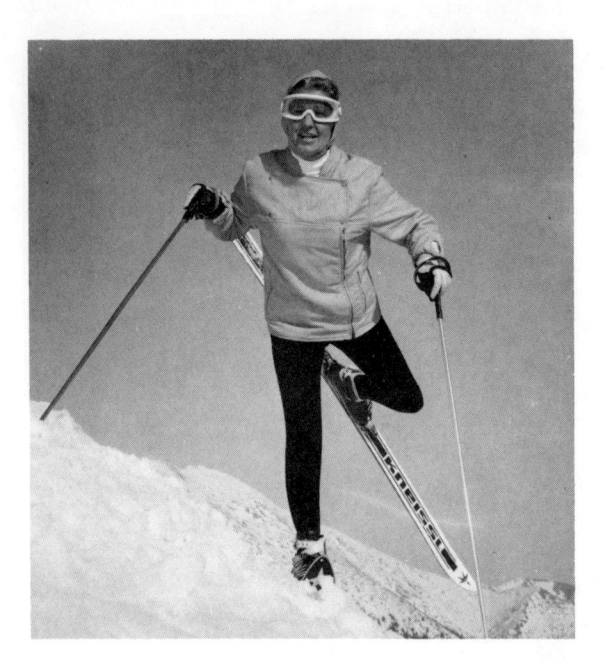

EXERCISE 61:
Lift one ski backward and up as high as you can. The quicker you do it, the better. This movement is also used when turning around in place.

you have already been practicing ski exercises for weeks beforehand, or completely forgot them, it is important now on the track to get yourself in shape by action! How much nicer it is to sweep over the slope, pleasantly tingling, than to go through the first few curves shivering and aching.

Try exercises without skis on your feet, some with skis on — and then you can go!

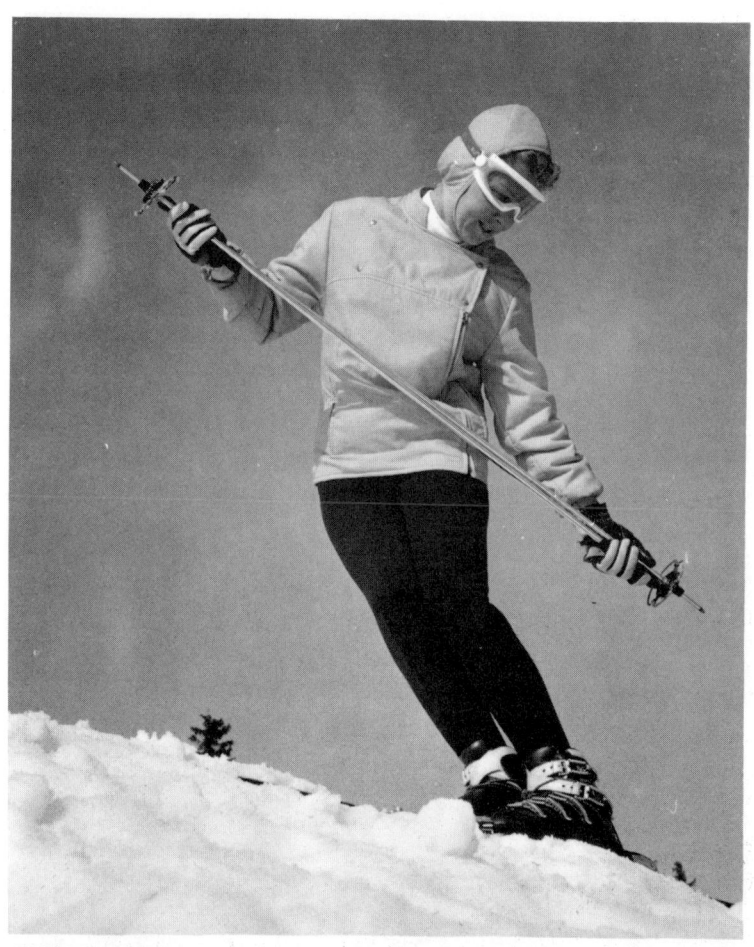

EXERCISE 62:
At an angle to the slope, put your weight on the uphill ski so your body weight is downhill. Bend your knees forward, turn your trunk towards the downslope, with pole ends held obliquely, and bend deeply backward. To complete the exercise, from an almost erect position, drop your body and at the same time press forward from the heels. This corresponds to the final phase of a swing.

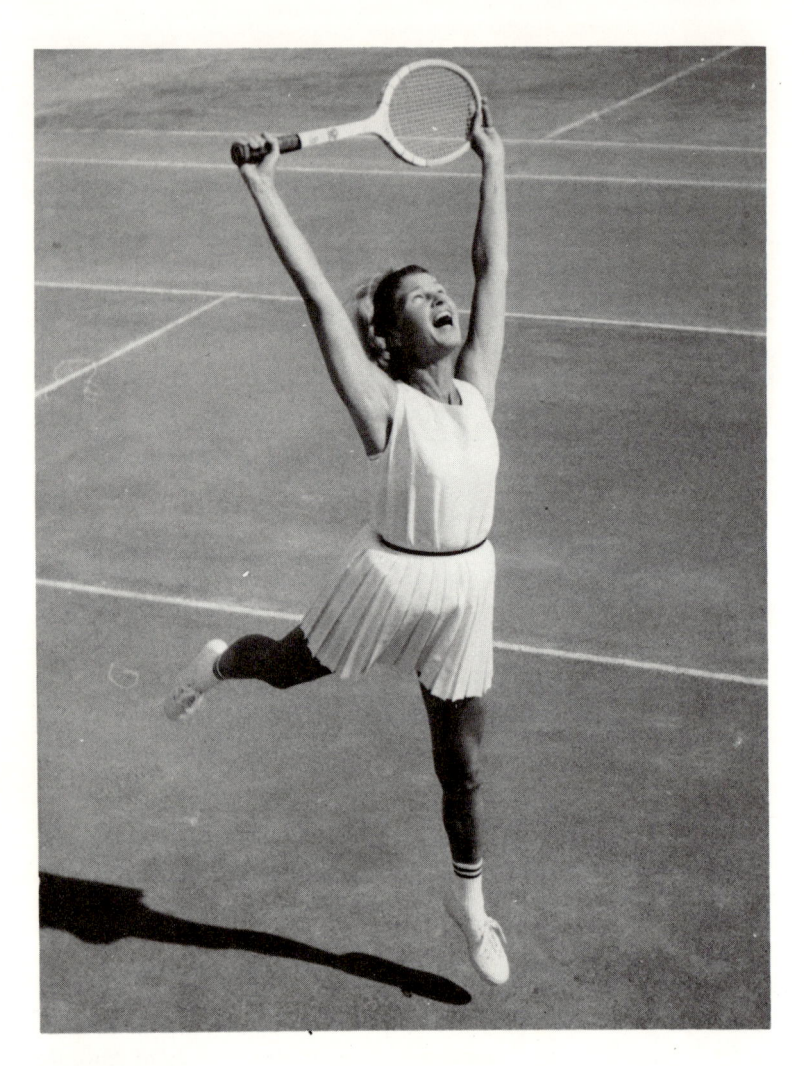

EXERCISE 63:
From a standing position, leap up with a flexible stretch upward of your whole body, raising one leg behind. Land in a standing position, relax, and let your body sag a little forward.

CONDITIONING FOR TENNIS

Are you in good enough condition to play tennis? Possibly not, for there is scarcely any other sport in which play, intense physical training, and grace are so ideally co-ordinated. You must be in tip-top shape, so overlook nothing in the way of conditioning. You will certainly suffer in the first hours of coping with tennis if you do!

Every sport requires preparatory training, and mastery of

EXERCISE 64:
For strengthening arms and legs, stand on a rung of the ladder of the umpire's tower. Hold on with one hand. Spring sideways, raising your free arm and leg quickly. Repeat the exercise with the other leg.

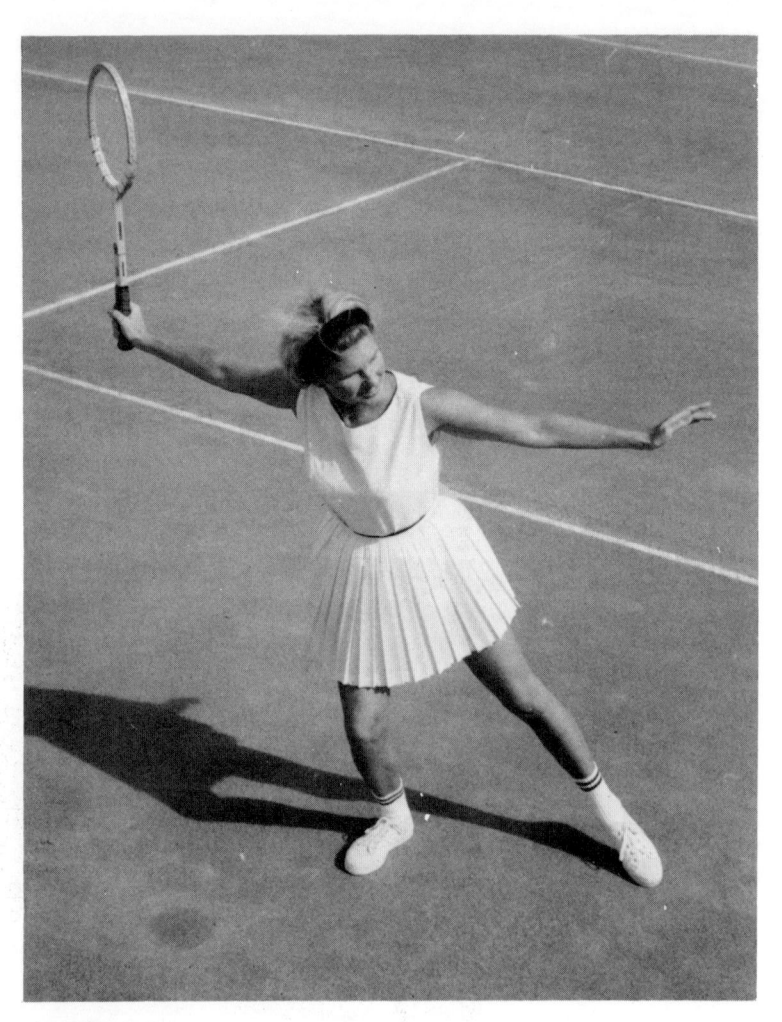

EXERCISE 65:
With feet apart, strike far out with a forehand stroke, shifting the weight of your body to your left leg and at the same time swinging powerfully through with your arm. Then swing back again and transfer the weight to your right leg.

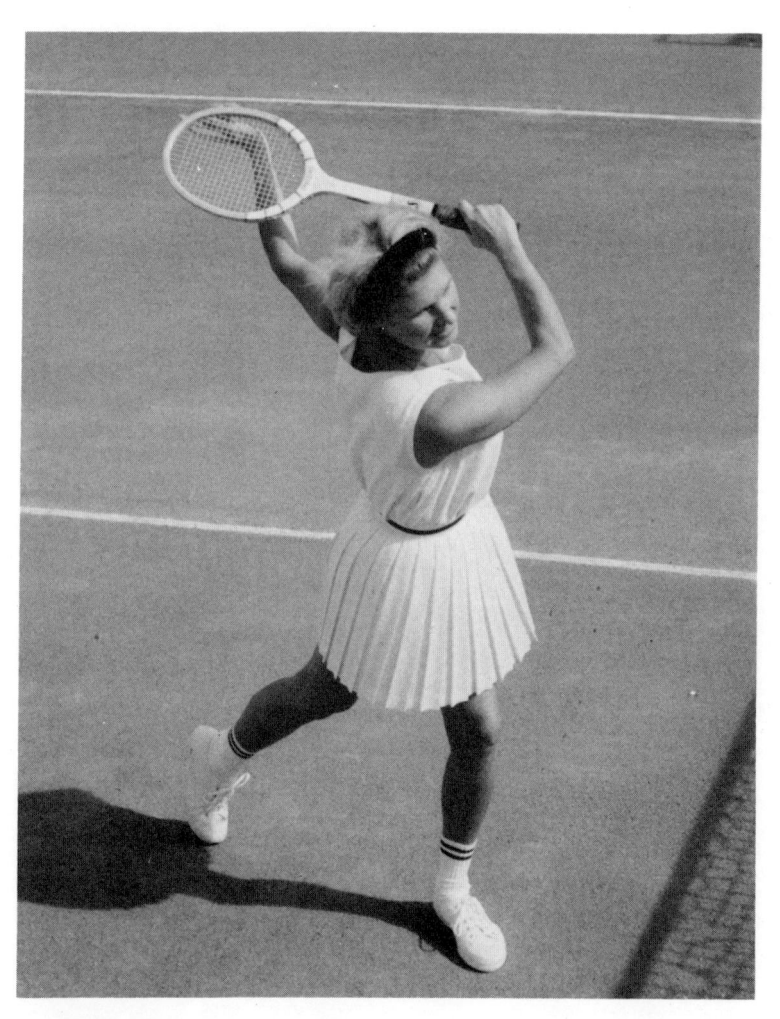

EXERCISE 66:
Turn your body over towards the left for a backhand stroke. Then strike far out and swing through to the right, shifting your weight to your right leg, then again back on your left leg and make another swing.

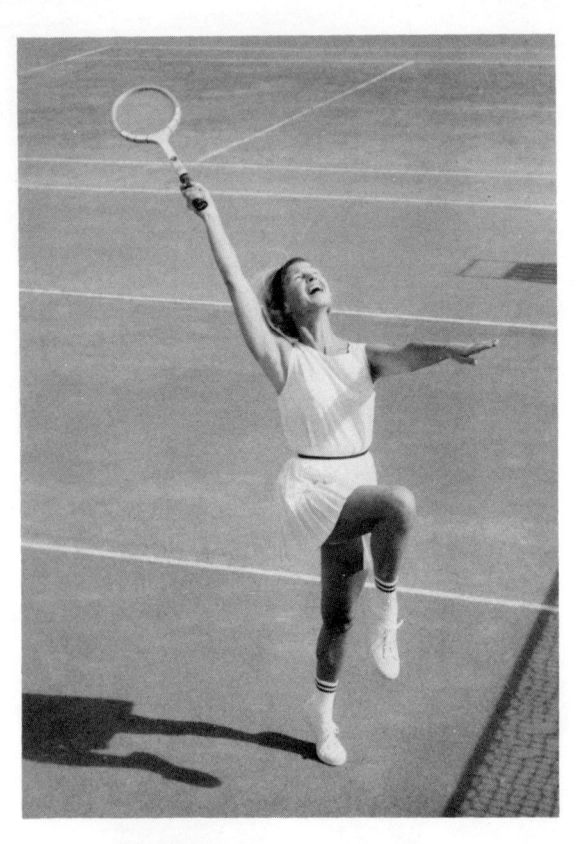

EXERCISE 67:
Spring up and swing the racket high behind you in a large, circular arm movement. At the same time, raise your right leg, then fall forward in a little lunge. This is excellent training for serving.

technique leads to real pleasure in any game, especially tennis. How do you achieve this mastery? By general body control, plenty of speed in your legs, endurance and energy in arms and shoulders, maneuverability, and the ability to react.

BEACH EXERCISES

Finally the wonderful beach season is here! Who doesn't enjoy thinking of hours of lazing on the beach in the summer or on a winter vacation in the South, where suntans are the order of the day and breezes sweep refreshingly over you. It is dangerous, however, to give yourself up to this lazy life, dangerous for both a slim figure and good disposition. A person cannot always just be splashing in the water or roasting in the sun; every now and again, one must move about a little. How would a few playful beach exercises grab you? Your swimming stroke will improve as your muscles develop

EXERCISE 68:
Sit, pass the ball under your left leg, then back under your right leg. If possible, do this exercise with both legs off the ground.

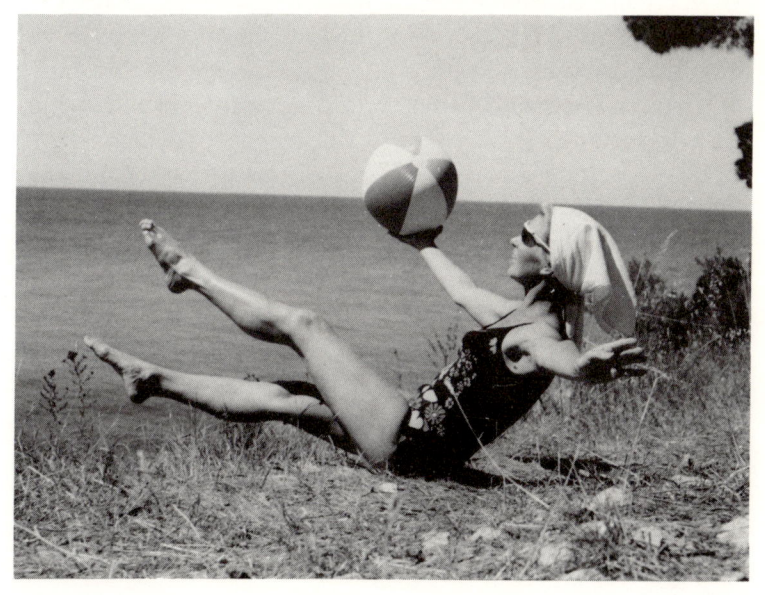

"tone" and your diving form will be admired as your legs and thighs lose their flabbiness. Swimming is perhaps the best exercise for getting your stomach flattened out.

Your children will be especially delighted, if their parents exercise and play with them. Your apparatus need only be a ball, a bath towel, a sun hat, or a jump rope. The most popular of all playthings is the wonderful, colorful water ball. You can exercise endlessly with it, throw it, roll it, catch it! If you come out of the water feeling a little chilly, a few vigorous moments with a ball will soon make you feel pleasantly warmed up!

Here are a few more tips for all beach vacationists! You will naturally want to make good use of the healing power of warm sand, so take long walks along the beach, barefooted of course! Every stride strengthens your foot muscles, since your toes have to grip firmly as you go. In this walk, you will be practicing the simplest and best foot exercise. For slim legs and firm thighs, run in shallow to knee-deep water! Running this way is made more difficult by the resistance the water sets up, and such exercise certainly makes the muscles work efficiently!

Not least, exercise provides a sureness of movement that results in a beautiful swimming stroke, a neat diving posture and a graceful walk.

EXERCISE 69:
Toss the ball up hard, stretching your entire body after it. Inhale. Catch it, inclining your torso slightly forward. Exhale.

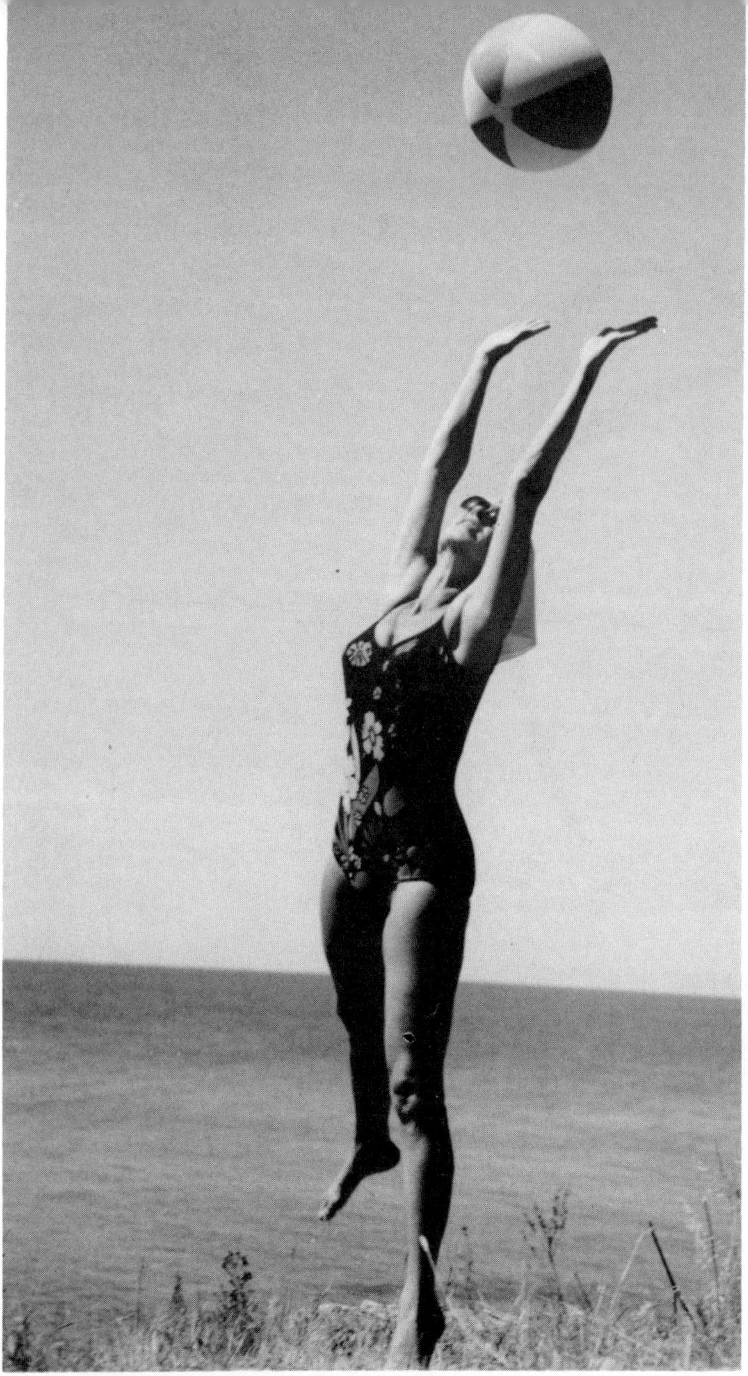

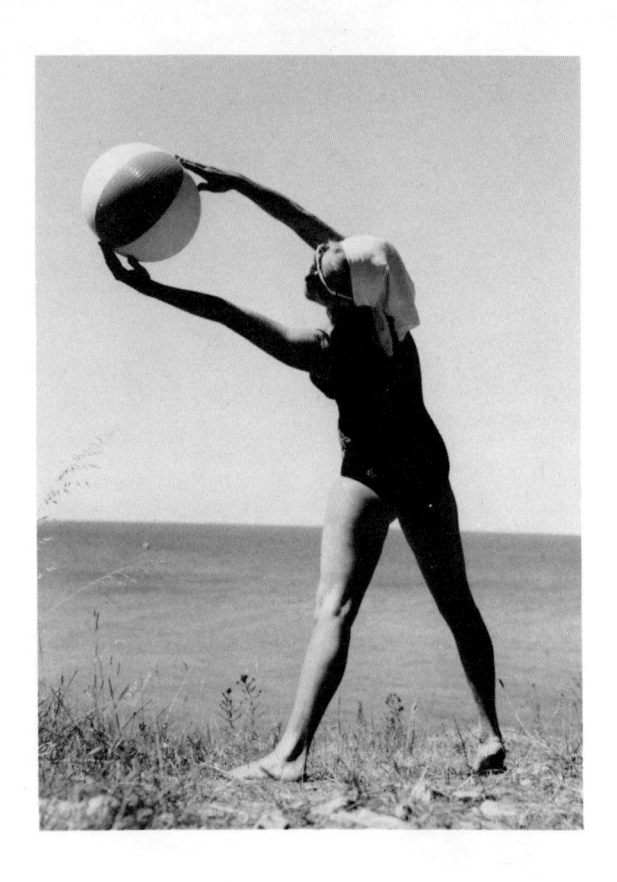

EXERCISE 70:
Holding the ball in your hands, swing your body in large circles, constantly alternating direction to keep from getting dizzy. This results in flexibility around the waist.

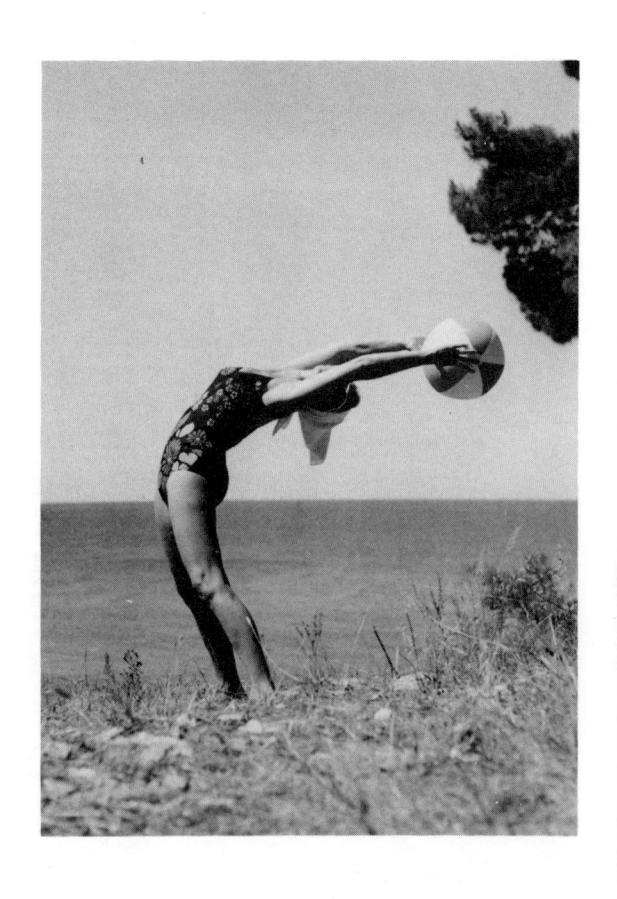

EXERCISE 71:
Spread your legs wide apart. Bend down far forward with the ball twice while exhaling. Straighten your body and bend over backward. Inhale.

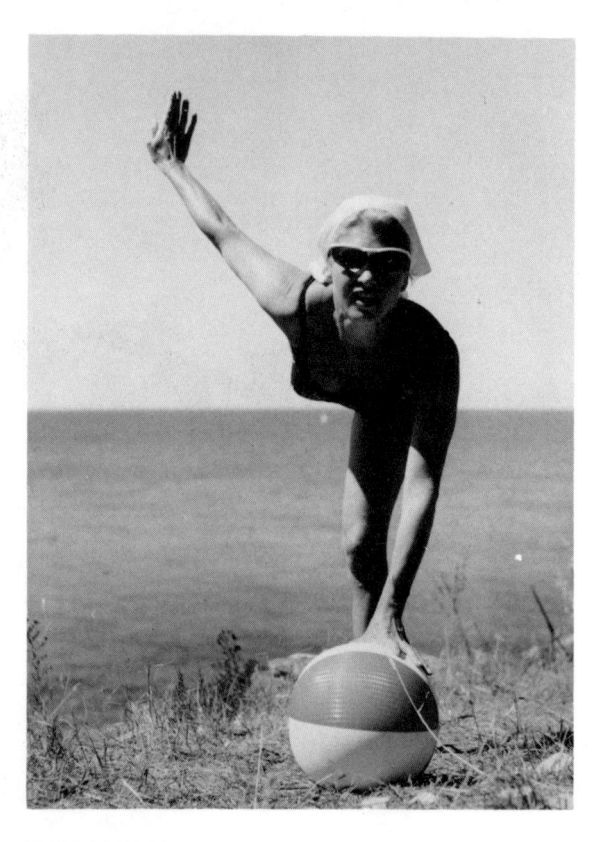

EXERCISE 72:
First stand erect, arms raised, and inhale. Then bend forward, support yourself on one hand on the ball and at the same time swing one leg back and up. Exhale. Next time, switch hands on the ball and hoist the other leg!

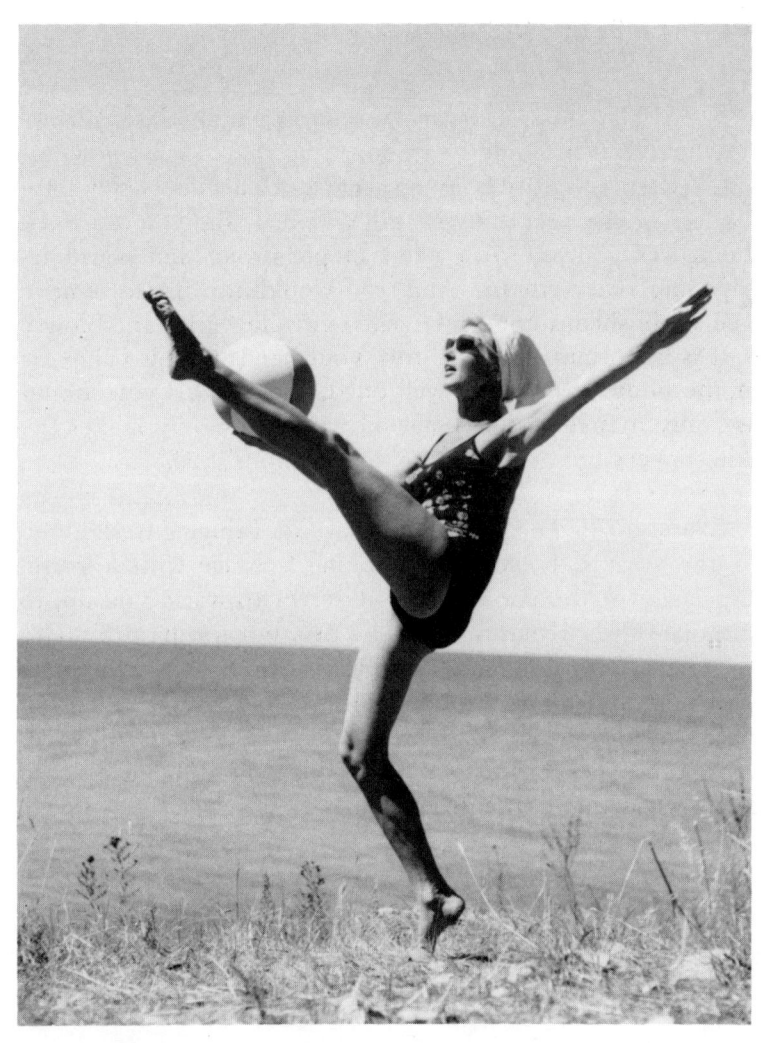

EXERCISE 73:
Swing one leg high, quickly pass the ball under it and receive it in the other hand. Then take two steps and swing the other leg high, repeating the ball pass.

A LITTLE SELF-MASSAGE

A first class masseuse (or masseur) is not always available. How practical it would be, then, to be able to massage yourself! Often an entire body massage is not needed; often only the legs or the neck muscles are cramped, and you can work them over yourself with a few simple stroke- and kneading-grips and relieve them. And who would not like to remove well established, stubborn fat pads with a few grips and blows?

It is important that not only your hands but also all parts of the body involved be well oiled, and for this you should use only a first-class massage-oil. This not only makes the skin slippery but at the same time well nourished.

Exercise 74: The simplest massage for bringing fresh blood to the area is, however, a stroking massage with a brush. Especially in the cool season, it serves to warm you up, to stimulate the circulation. Take a dry, not too hard but also not too soft, brush in hand and pass it with light pressure over your legs and arms, stroking toward your heart. Brush in circles over your abdomen and hips, until the skin turns red. As a consequence you will feel a pleasant, tingling flow of fresh blood that will enliven you.

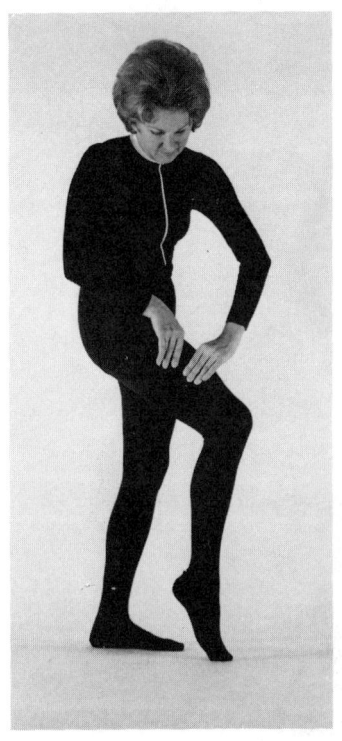

EXERCISE 75:
Upper thigh. Take the relaxed muscle between thumb and fingers and grip deeply while thoroughly kneading. However, don't pinch with your fingertips alone, but grab hold vigorously with your entire hand. Also, work over your hip area in the same way, and don't forget the inner side of your thigh.

EXERCISE 76:
Hips. Press with both fists and describe circles left and right. After a long period of sitting still, massage of these areas is immediately necessary.

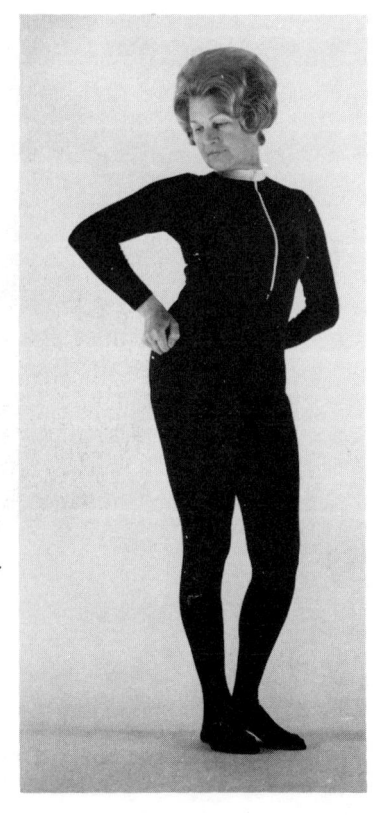

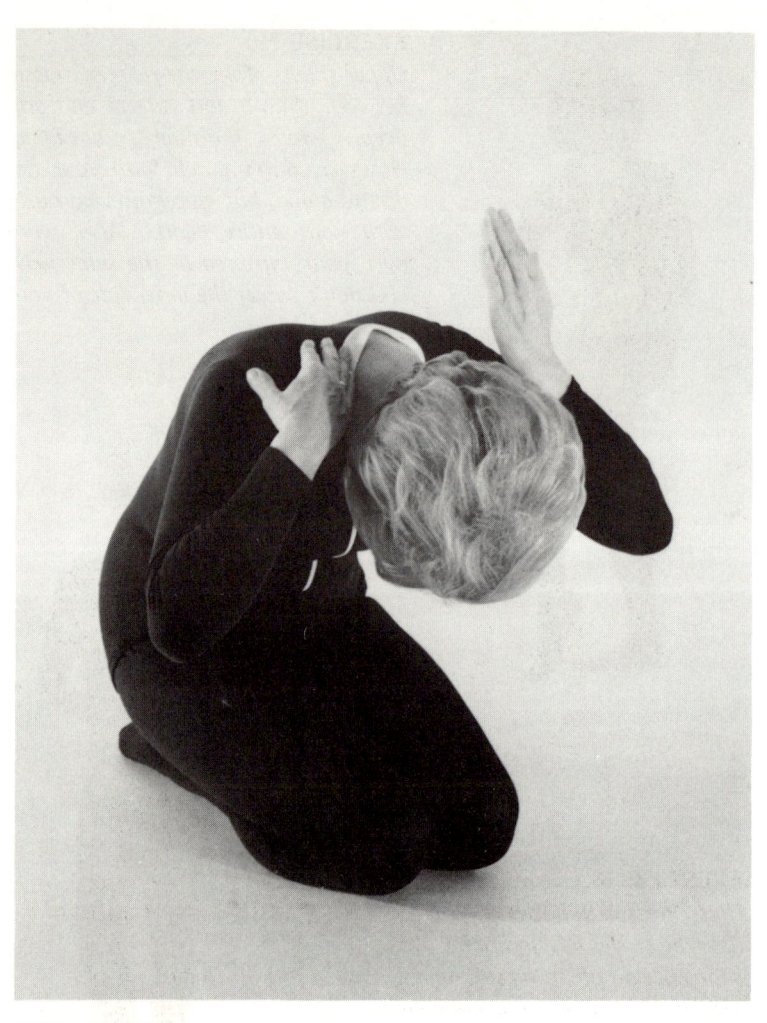

EXERCISE 77:
Neck. First thump your neck muscles with your palms and thus enliven them. A stiff head position, for instance, when typing or sewing, leads to cramping, so that headaches often result. This will prevent them.

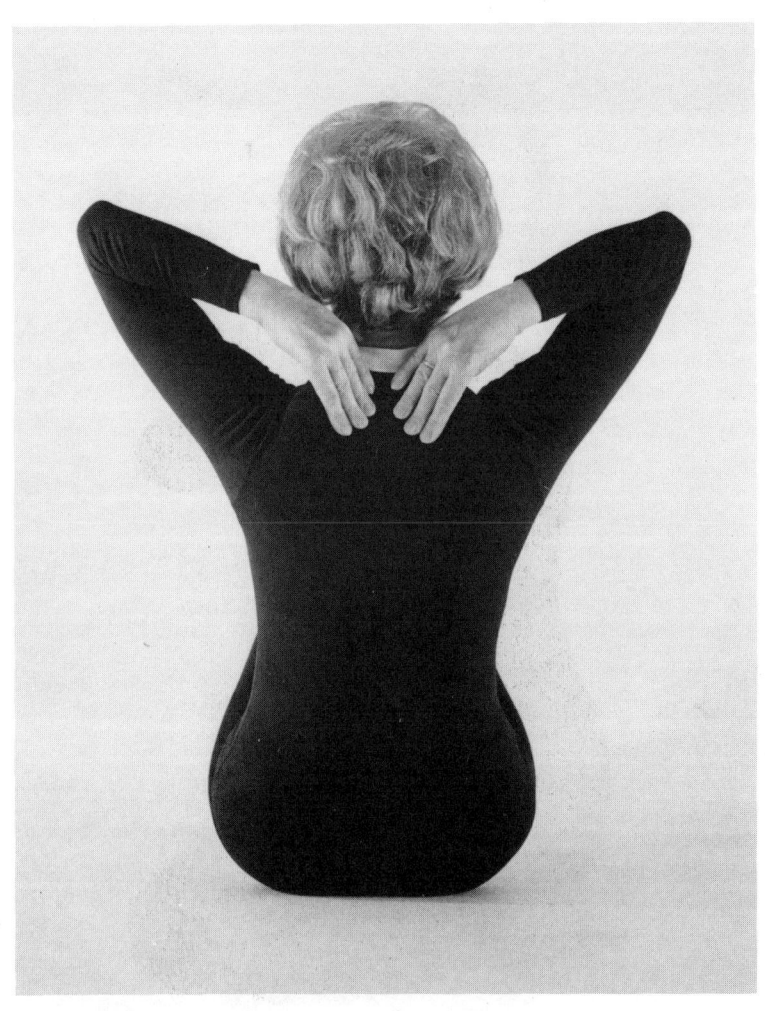

EXERCISE 78:
This massage, too, enlivens the region around the neck and expels excess fat. Place hands on neck as shown, so that your thumbs point forward and your fingers back. Now grip deeply and knead thoroughly, pressing the muscle upward towards your neck.

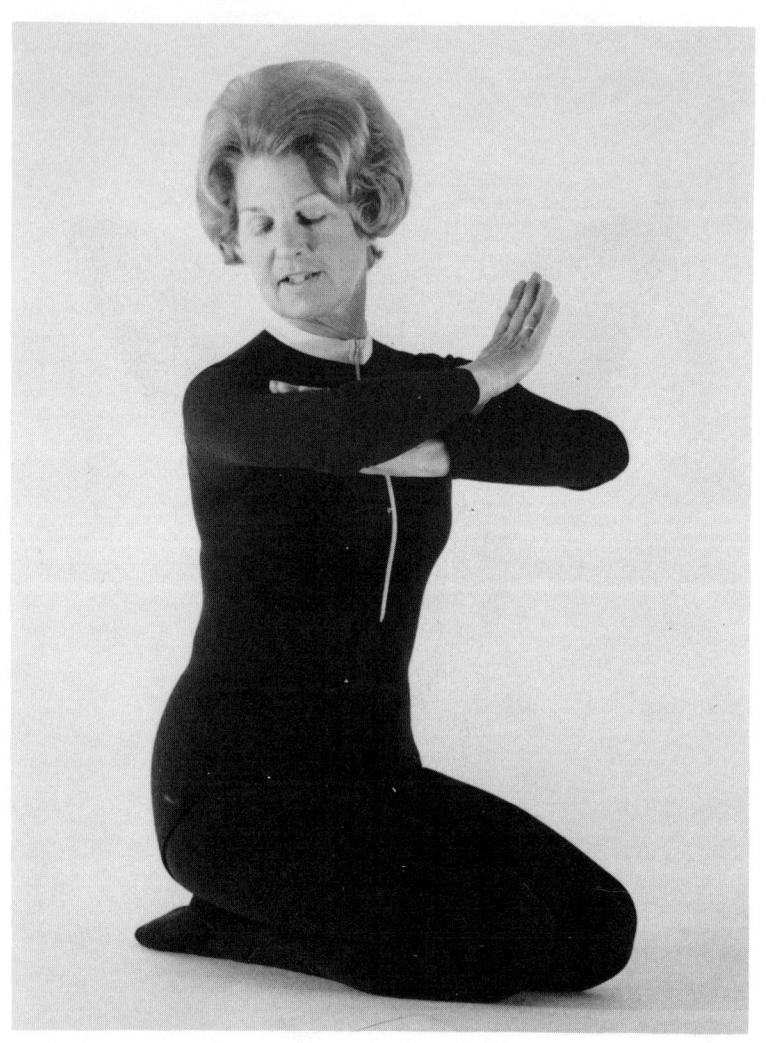

EXERCISE 79:
Upper arms. Cross your forearms and knead and pound your upper arms to stir up circulation. Flabby upper arms are ugly and hurt when tight or cramped.

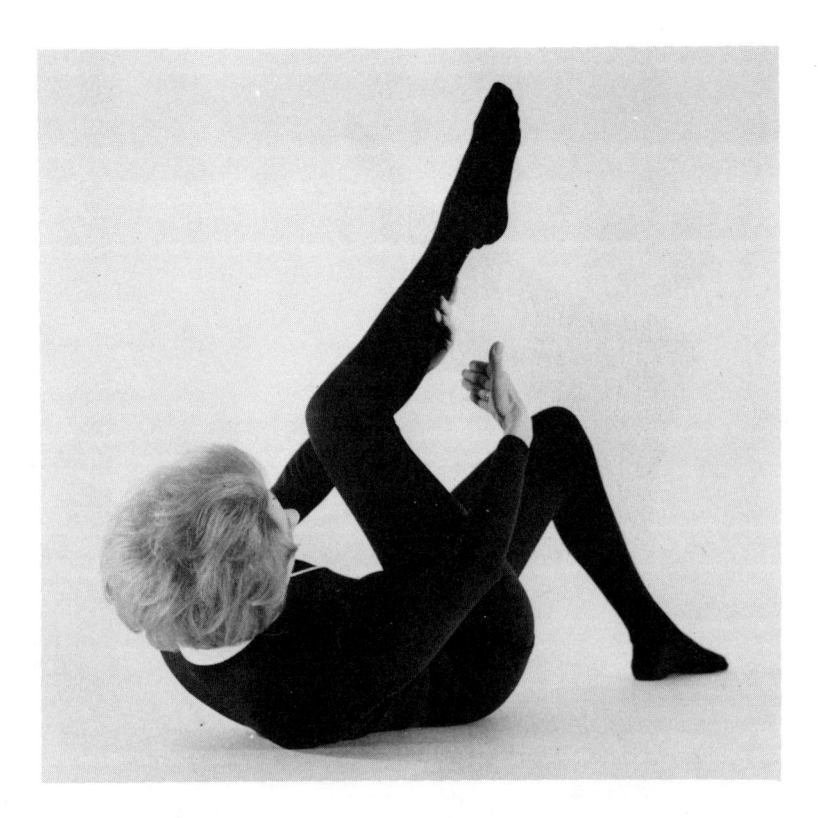

EXERCISE 80:
Legs. Hold one leg up loosely and pound the calf from left and right, thus enlivening the muscle. Standing still for long stretches is especially hard on the legs.

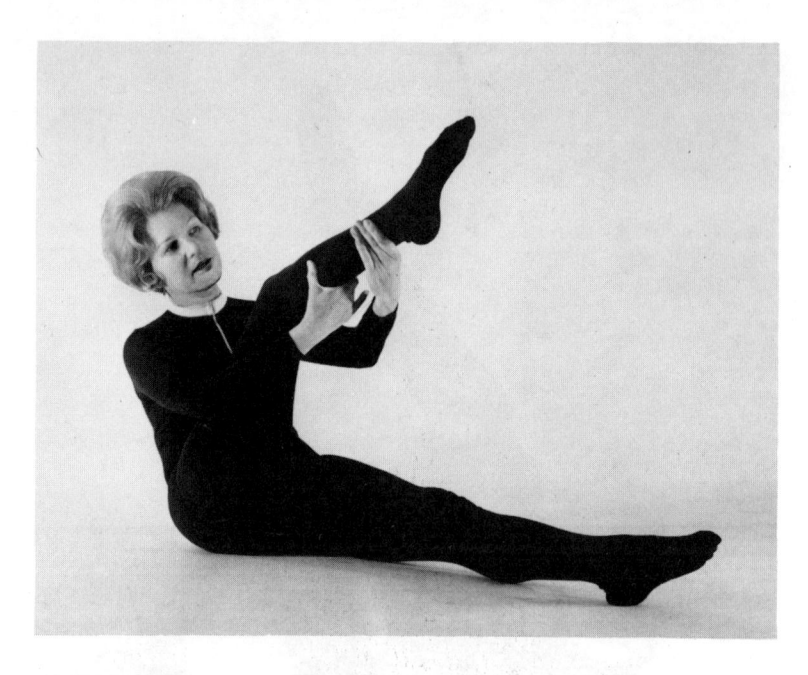

EXERCISE 81:
Stroke the loose calf-muscle from your ankle upwards toward your knee, as if it might have slipped downward and you are now pushing it back into its proper place.

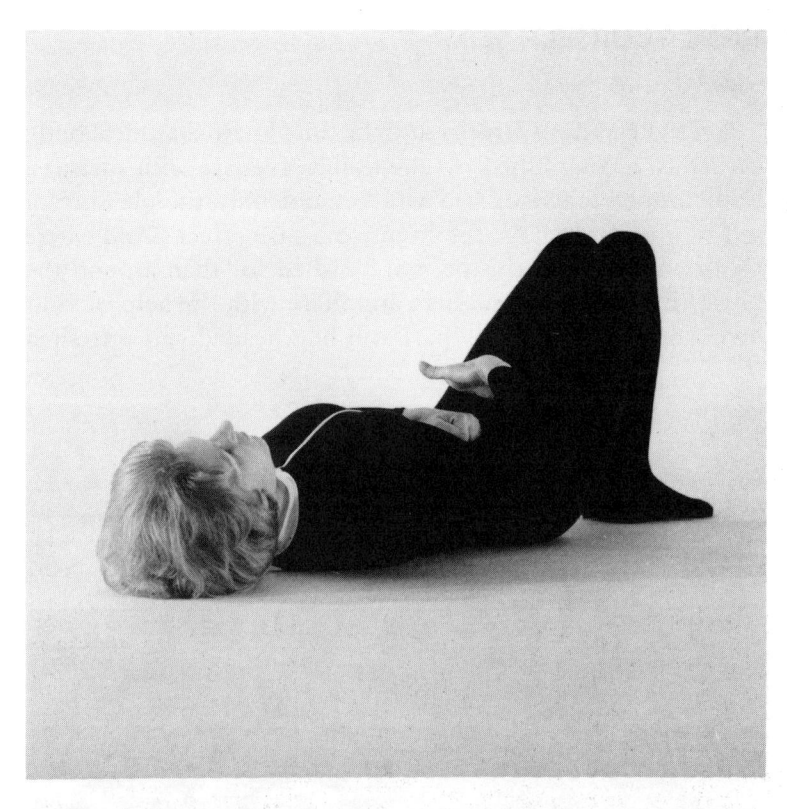

EXERCISE 82:
To bring about a slim figure, but also to get rid of a flabby tummy and/or digestive trouble, an intense massage grip on the abdominal muscles is a great help. First enliven by pounding — as in working over the leg and neck muscles — then lay one fist on your belly, the other hand flat upon it, and now, applying pressure, move your hands around in circles. Do this exercise lying on your back, for that way the abdominal muscles can be relaxed the best.

ROLL YOURSELF SLIM

Even the ancient Greeks in their time knew that ideal body care was accomplished by combining exercise with massage. With proper practice, you will get not only the pleasure of self-movement but also an intense massage effect. And where on the body could this be more wished for than around the hips? By rolling around here and there with the help of your own body weight, every part will be kneaded and refreshed

EXERCISE 83:
"Bicycle," but in doing so, roll back and forth, keeping your legs up off the floor. Let your hands remain firmly planted on the floor.

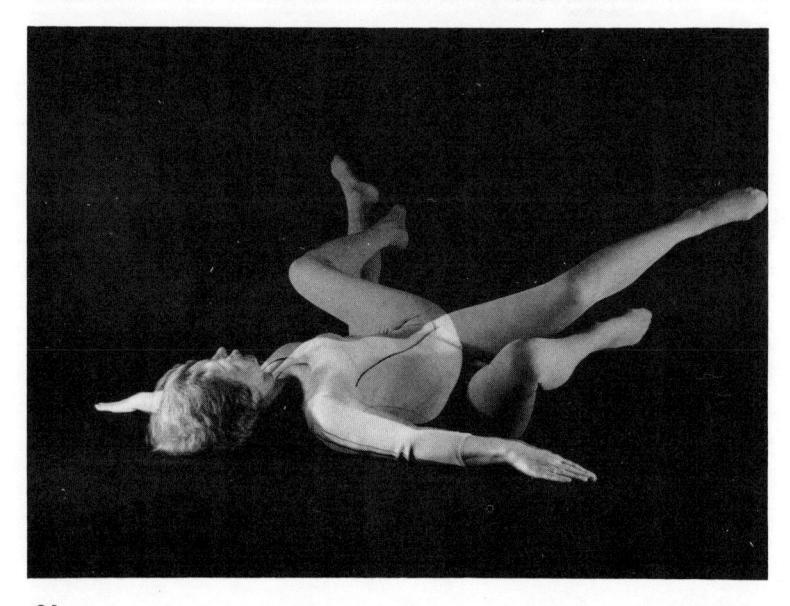

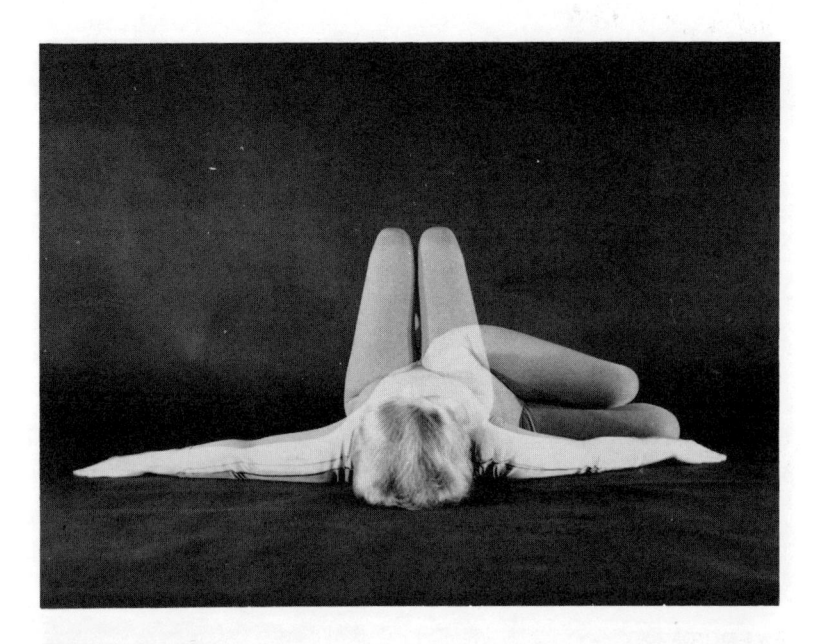

EXERCISE 84:
Lie on your back, legs drawn up. Let your two legs fall to the floor, first to the left, then to the right. The louder your muscles clatter on the floor, the more effective the massage action. Let your feet remain in place throughout.

with a tingling flow of blood. These exercises are in no way difficult. Your whole body is exercised, your waist made supple and your movements graceful.

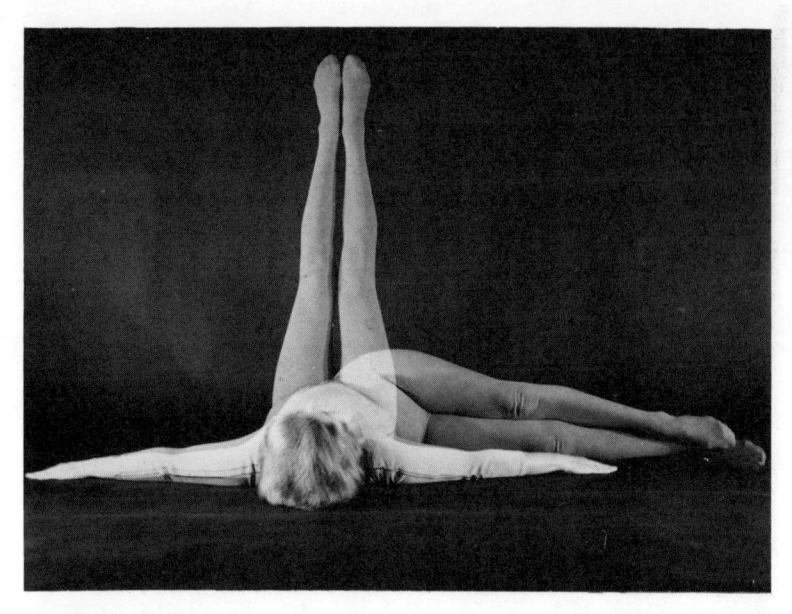

EXERCISE 85:
Stretch out both legs and raise them straight up, then let them sink to the floor, first on one side, then on the other, like a windshield wiper, but don't let them hit the floor hard. Exhale as you raise your legs; that makes it easier.

A FINAL WORD

Now that you have drilled through many exercises, you should have found precisely the right thing for you. Ski holidays are at hand, a golf game is in the offing, you have a chance to enter a tennis tournament, or some friends have invited you to their pool. You want your body to be in shape — and if you have been exercising daily, it will be.

Perhaps your sports schedule has been stimulated by this

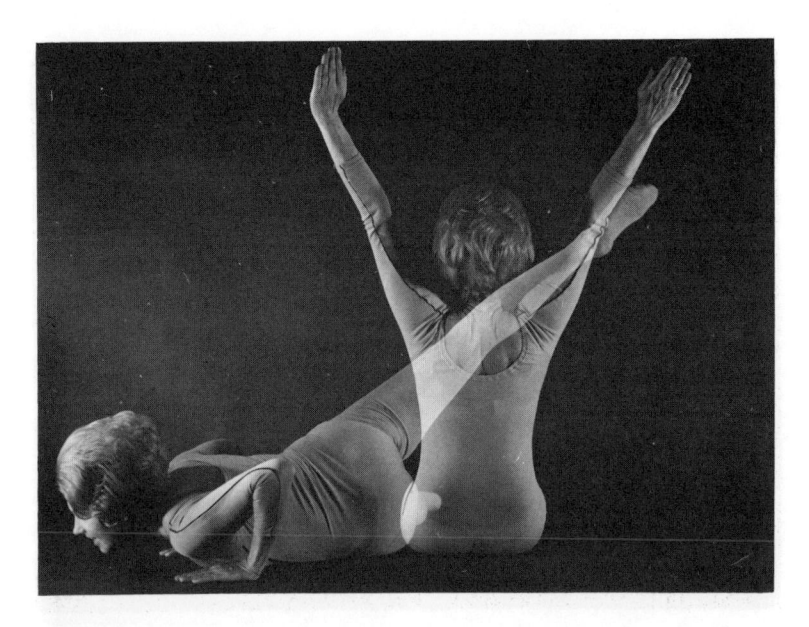

EXERCISE 86:
While in a sitting position, fall over to the left, letting your torso sink down deeply, and at the same time swing your right leg up high. Then push yourself back up, coming to an erect sitting position. Next fall over to the right, and repeat.

"picture book." Perhaps you have succeeded in moving into an entirely new schedule for your spare time, and are making your days richer and your life more healthy. Hopefully you are getting greater fulfilment in the joy of living through exercise.

How often I have heard this observation from old and young: "Since I have taken up exercise, I am an entirely new person!" Or: "If I can't exercise on Friday evening, the whole weekend is ruined for me!"

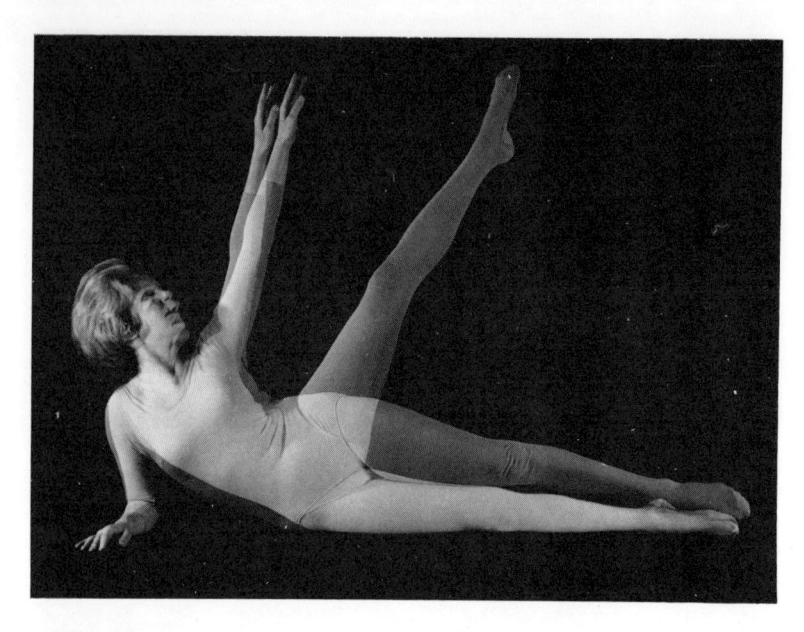

EXERCISE 87:
Lie on your side, supporting yourself on your right forearm. Swing your left leg high towards your raised hand and let it back down again with a controlled movement. Practice this ten times on each side.

Although you have gone through 90 exercises, there is still a lot more to be said. This book is meant to be a good beginning, an introduction. All the exercises are significant and easy to understand; the photos are to inspire you and point the way to doing it right.

Still one more request: Exercise is not accomplished in two minutes. Exercise does not consist of a few knee-bends to wake you up. Everyone should exercise methodically, even in the shortest practice session. Begin only somewhat energetically, revivifying your whole body; follow this with

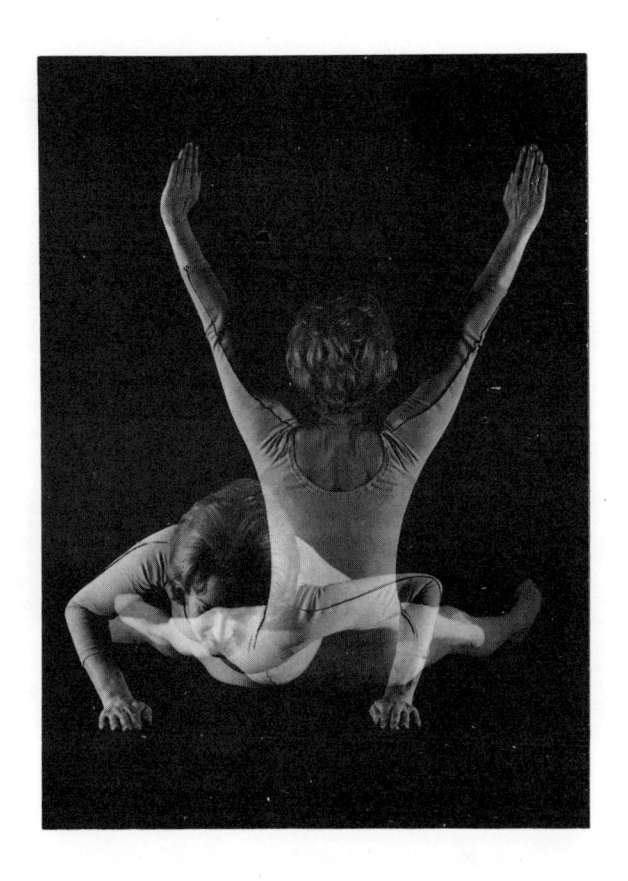

EXERCISE 88:
In sitting position with legs spread wide apart, turn your hips vigorously backward towards the left, supporting yourself on your hands against the floor. In this position, let your body down deeply, with your legs remaining in place. Then vigorously push yourself back up, sit up straight as before, then turn backwards to the right and repeat.

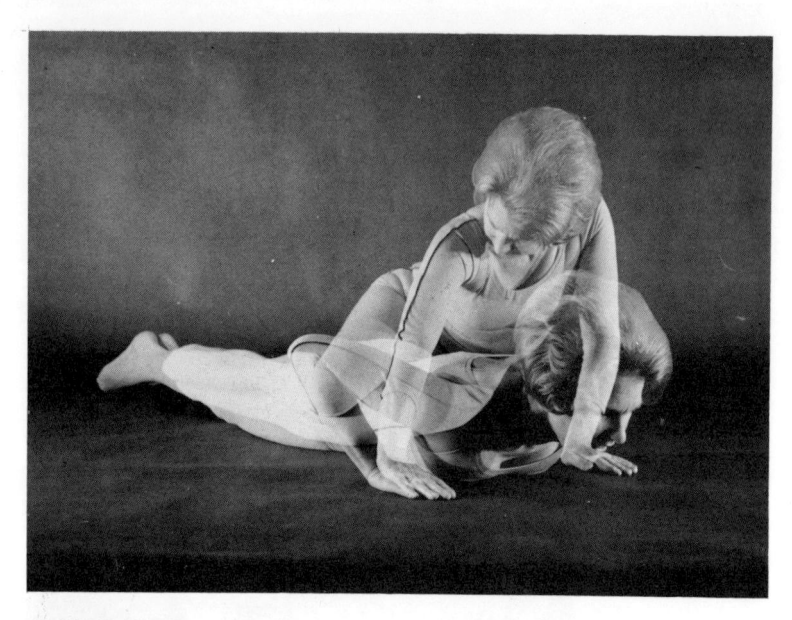

EXERCISE 89:
Lie on your stomach, hands pressing the floor under your shoulders. Press your torso up high, at the same time rolling to one side on your hip and draw one knee upward toward your trunk. Exhale as you do this. Now, stretch your legs out straight. Let your trunk sink back to starting position.

the special training exercises for sports and at the end, without fail, relax and deep breathe! And should you have time for no more than three exercises, then take special note of the following:

1. Warm up first; stimulate your circulation!
2. Go into your special needs; for example, foot exercise or hip-roll exercise.
3. Wind up with vigorous breathing and relaxing exercises.

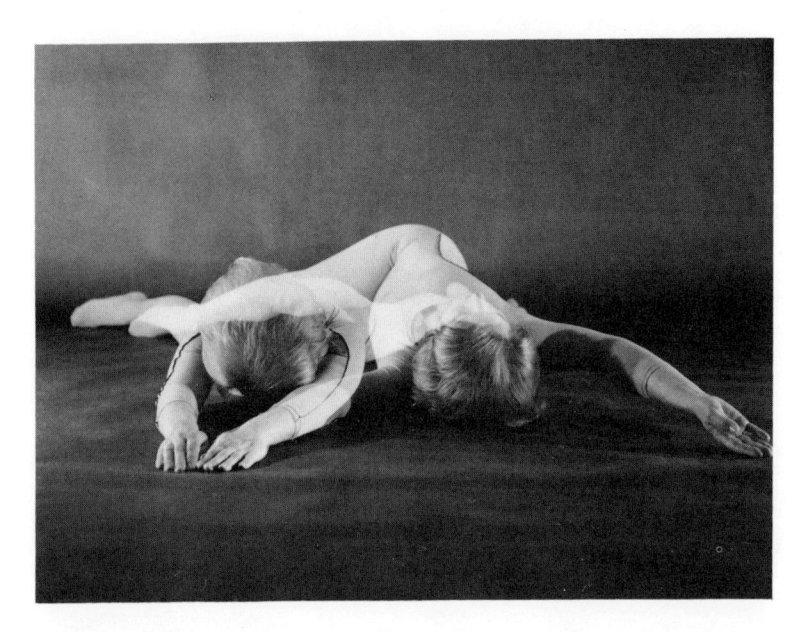

EXERCISE 90:
Lie on your stomach, legs spread wide apart, the wider the better, for that way the turning effect on your waist will be greater. Stretch your arms out over your head, palms against the floor. Raise your right arm, turn your torso towards the back, until your hand touches the floor. Inhale as you do this. Turn back to the starting position and exhale. Then turn to the left, and repeat.

INDEX

arms, upper, massaging 82

back
    aligning 36
    counteracting a rigid 35
    strengthening and
      straightening 12-13
beach, exercising on the 71-77
breasts, firming 14-15
breathing and stretching,
    exercise for 45

calf muscle, massaging 84
children, exercises for 49-52
circulation, stimulating 46-47

hips
    limbering 46-47
    massaging 79
    rolling on 86-87, 88, 89,
      90, 91, 92, 93
    slenderizing 7

legs
    conditioning 34, 35
    massaging 83, 84
limbering up 44-48

massage 78-85

muscle toning 20-22

neck, massaging 80-81

posture, correcting 16, 38-43, 48

relaxation, exercises for 19, 30-31

sitters, exercises for all-day 20, 21, 22, 23-24
skiing, conditioning for 53-66
sportsman, exercises for 32-37
standers, exercises for all-day 25-29
stomach muscles
    firming 8-9
    massaging 85
swayback, eliminating 12-13

tennis, conditioning for 67-70
thighs
    firming 17-18
    upper, massaging 79

waistline
    elasticity of 46
    slimming 10-11
    suppleness around 34-35